RE TOPICS IN PERIOPERATIVE MEDICINE

CORE TOPICS IN PERIOPERATIVE MEDICINE

by
Jonathan Hudsmith BM FRCA
Department of Anaesthesia
Peterborough Hospitals NHS Trust

Dan Wheeler MA BM BCh MRCP FRCA
Clinical Lecturer in Anaesthesia
University of Cambridge

Arun Gupta MA MBBS FRCA
Director of Postgraduate Medical Education
University of Cambridge

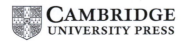
CAMBRIDGE
UNIVERSITY PRESS

CAMBRIDGE UNIVERSITY PRESS
Cambridge, New York, Melbourne, Madrid, Cape Town, Singapore, São Paulo, Delhi

Cambridge University Press
The Edinburgh Building, Cambridge CB2 8RU, UK

www.cambridge.org
Information on this title:www.cambridge.org/9780521730686

Published in the United States of America by Cambridge University Press, New York

First Published 2004
Reprinted by Cambridge University Press 2008

Printed in the United Kingdom at the University Press, Cambridge

A catalogue record for this publication is available from the British Library

ISBN 978-0-521-73068-6 paperback

Contents

Preface

Undergraduate medical education is continuously changing to meet the requirements for the training of future medical practitioners. Over the last few years the concept of perioperative medicine has evolved encompassing the preoperative assessment and optimisation of patients, the intraoperative and postoperative management of these patients and importantly the recognition, diagnosis and treatment of the critically ill patient. The relevance of this to undergraduate medical students is undeniable and a number of medical schools have now incorporated a module of Perioperative Medicine into their curricula for medical students.

The aims of this book are to provide concise, informative chapters on many aspects of perioperative medicine, allowing medical students to bridge the gap between their clinical attachment in this specialty, first year house officer jobs and preparation for postgraduate examinations. We make no apology for repeating important messages and subsequently there may be some crossover of subject matter between chapters.

Changes to the structure of Senior House Officer training will result in incorporation of a Foundation year for the majority of newly qualified doctors. This book covers many of the situations and problems that these doctors will have to face. By providing a broad overview of the perioperative period, this text can be a very useful quick reference guide.

Effectively caring for patients in the perioperative period is a complex and demanding job. Doctors and nurses need to be able to detect early signs of any problems during this time, so that interventions can be planned to optimise outcome for their patients. This book should help staff achieve this goal.

This book will also be useful to those preparing for Surgical, Anaesthetic and Accident and Emergency postgraduate examinations. Nurses and other healthcare professionals, who are taking on increasing clinical responsibilities within the perioperative period, will also find this book invaluable.

Jonathan Hudsmith
Dan Wheeler
Arun Gupta

August 2003

Contributors

Sue Abdy MBBS DRCOG FRCA
Department of Anaesthesia
Queen Elizabeth Hospital, King's Lynn

Mark Abrahams MBChB DA FRCA
Department of Anaesthesia
Norfolk & Norwich University Hospital NHS Trust

Ian Bridgland MBBS MSc DRCOG FRCA FANZCA
Department of Anaesthesia
St. Vincent's Hospital, Sydney, Australia

Tim Clarke MBChB FRCA
Department of Anaesthesia
Blackburn Royal Infirmary

Warren Fisher MBChB FRCA
Department of Anaesthesia
Royal Berkshire Hospital, Reading

Simon Fletcher MBBS FRCA
Department of Anaesthesia
Norfolk & Norwich University Hospital NHS Trust

Wendy Gatling MBChB DM FRCP
Department of Medicine & Diabetes Centre
Poole Hospital NHS Trust

Andy Gregg BM MRCP FRCA
Neurocritical Care Unit
Addenbrooke's NHS Trust, Cambridge

Arun Gupta MA MBBS FRCA
Director of Postgraduate Medical Education
University of Cambridge

Jonathan Hudsmith BM FRCA
Department of Anaesthesia
Peterborough Hospitals NHS Trust

Paul Hughes MBChB FRCA
Department of Anaesthesia
Peterborough Hospitals NHS Trust

Andrew Johnston MA MB BChir FRCA
Department of Anaesthesia
Addenbrooke's NHS Trust, Cambridge

Jeremy Lermitte BM FRCA
Department of Anaesthesia
Addenbrooke's NHS Trust, Cambridge

Michael Lindop MA MB BChir FRCA
Department of Anaesthesia
Addenbrooke's NHS Trust, Cambridge

Iain MacKenzie DM MRCP FRCA
Department of Anaesthesia
Addenbrooke's NHS Trust, Cambridge

John McNamara MBBS FRCA
Department of Anaesthesia
Bedford Hospital

Mike Masding MBBS MRCP
Department of Medicine & Diabetes Centre
Poole Hospital NHS Trust

Quentin Milner MBChB FRCA
Department of Anaesthesia
Queen Alexandra Hospital, Portsmouth

Fraz Mir BSc MBBS MRCP
Department of Intensive Care
Addenbrooke's NHS Trust, Cambridge

Vilas Navapurkar MBChB DA FRCA
Department of Anaesthesia
Addenbrooke's NHS Trust, Cambridge

Richard Neal MA MB BChir
Department of Paediatrics
Kings Mill Hospital, Mansfield

Mike Palmer BPharm PhD MBBS FRCA
Department of Anaesthesia
West Suffolk Hospital, Bury St. Edmunds

Karen Pedersen MBBCh FANZCA
Department of Anaesthesia
Auckland Hospital, New Zealand

Parameswaran Pillai MD FRCA
Department of Anaesthesia
Addenbrooke's NHS Trust, Cambridge

Anand Sardesai MBBS MD DA FRCA
Department of Anaesthesia
Addenbrooke's NHS Trust, Cambridge

Christopher Sharpe MBBS FRCA
Department of Anaesthesia
Norfolk & Norwich University Hospital NHS Trust

Helen Smith MBBS FRCA
Department of Anaesthesia
Addenbrooke's NHS Trust, Cambridge

Dan Wheeler MA BM BCh MRCP FRCA
Clinical Lecturer in Anaesthesia
University of Cambridge

Ingrid Wilkins BSc FRCA
Department of Anaesthesia
Addenbrooke's NHS Trust, Cambridge

Katrina Williams BSc MBChB FRCA
Department of Anaesthesia
Norfolk & Norwich University Hospital NHS Trust

Peter Young MD FRCA
Department of Anaesthesia
Queen Elizabeth Hospital, King's Lynn

Perioperative management of cardiovascular disease

John McNamara

Introduction

Cardiovascular disease is common in the surgical population, occurring in at least 10% of patients presenting for surgery. Their assessment can be broadly divided into consideration of the following:

1. Ischaemic heart disease
2. Hypertension
3. Cardiac failure
4. Cardiac arrhythmias and pacemakers
5. Valvular disease

The reason for assessing patients before surgery is to:

1. Make an estimate of their risk of cardiovascular morbidity and mortality
2. Make a plan to investigate and intervene to optimise the patient's condition if possible
3. Plan the operation and anaesthetic technique
4. Arrange appropriate postoperative monitoring and treatment

Assessment via history, examination and investigations

History should particularly focus on the patient's functional ability. The American College of Cardiology and American Heart Foundation have devised a method of assessing function by means of simple questions about activity, and quantified the physiological reserve required to attain certain levels of activity using 'metabolic equivalent tasks (METs)' (Table 1.1).

It is also important to consider:

- any previous admissions with cardiac conditions
- exercise limits, on the flat and up stairs (e.g. how many flights?)
- precipitants and frequency of angina, frequency of use of nitrate spray or tablets
- symptoms of cardiac failure – paroxysmal nocturnal dyspnoea, ankle oedema
- if hypertensive, history of control/previous readings
- pacemakers – type, recent checks and indication for insertion

Examination should include a full cardiovascular assessment and blood pressure. Investigations will follow local guidelines, in particular an ECG should be ordered for any patient with cardiovascular disease and a chest X-ray ordered for any patient with cardiac related respiratory symptoms. Most murmurs will require an echocardiogram. An echocardiogram is also useful to assess moderate to severe heart failure.

Table 1.1 Estimated energy requirements for various activities

1 MET	4 METs
■ Can you take care of yourself?	■ Climb a flight of stairs or walk up a hill?
■ Eat, dress, or use the toilet?	■ Walk on level ground at 4 mph or 6.4 km/h?
■ Walk indoors around the house?	■ Run a short distance?
■ Walk a block or two on level ground at 2–3 mph or 3.2–4.8 km/h?	■ Do heavy work around the house like scrubbing floors or lifting or moving heavy furniture?
4 METs ■ Do light work around the house like dusting or washing dishes?	■ Participate in moderate recreational activities like golf, bowling, dancing, doubles tennis, or throwing a baseball or football?
	>10 METs ■ Participate in strenuous sports like swimming, singles tennis, football, basketball, or skiing?

MET indicates metabolic equivalent.
Adapted from the Duke Activity Status Index (Hlatky MA, Boineau RE, Higginbotham MB, Lee KL, Mark DB, Califf RM, Cobb FR, Proyr DB. A brief self-administered questionnaire to determine functional capacity [the Duke Activity Status Index]. Am J Cardiol 1989; 64: 651–654) and AHA Exercise Standards (Fletcher GF, Balady G, Froelicher VF, Hartley LH, Haskell WL, Pollock ML. Exercise standards: A statement for healthcare professionals from the American Heart Association. Circulation 1995; 91: 580–615).

Findings of concern/liaise with anaesthetist

1. myocardial infarct (MI) within the past 6 months

2. unstable/increasing angina

3. poorly treated cardiac failure (unable to lie flat with 2 pillows)

4. severe exercise limitation – symptoms on less than ordinary activity

5. untreated cardiac arrhythmias

6. systolic blood pressure >200 mmHg, diastolic blood pressure >100 mmHg

7. murmurs without a recent echocardiogram

1

Cardiac risk and surgery

Surgery stresses the cardiovascular system, the extent depending on a patient's age, urgency of surgery, site of surgery and length of surgery. The American College of Cardiology and American Heart Foundation have stratified cardiac event risk for non-cardiac surgery (Table 1.2).

Cardiac risk and anaesthesia

Anaesthesia also poses a significant stress to the cardiovascular system. The important risk factors for perioperative cardiac morbidity and mortality were identified by Goldman as long ago as the 1970s (Table 1.3). This index has a high specificity but low sensitivity, in other words it correctly identifies those at high risk by their high score but does not identify all high risk patients. Subsequent revisions and modifications have been made, but the Goldman index is still widely used to assess postoperative cardiac risk.

Table 1.2 Cardiac event risk* stratification for non-cardiac surgical procedures

High	Intermediate	Low†
(Reported cardiac risk often >5%)	(Reported cardiac risk generally <5%)	(Reported cardiac risk generally <1%)
■ Emergent major operations, particularly in the elderly	■ Intraperitoneal and intrathoracic surgery	■ Endoscopic procedures
■ Aortic and other major vascular surgery	■ Carotid endarterectomy surgery	■ Superficial procedures
■ Peripheral vascular surgery	■ Head and neck surgery	■ Cataract surgery
■ Anticipated prolonged surgical procedures associated with large fluid shifts and/or blood loss	■ Orthopedic surgery	■ Breast surgery
	■ Prostate surgery	

*Combined incidence of cardiac death and non-fatal myocardial infarction.
†Further preoperative cardiac testing is not generally required.

Table 1.3 **Goldman cardiac risk index**

Finding	Score
Evidence of uncontrolled cardiac failure, e.g. third heart sound, elevated jugulovenous pressure	11
Myocardial infarction within 6 months	10
Ventricular ectopic beats on ECG	7
Cardiac rhythm other than sinus	7
Age >70 years	5
Emergency surgery	4
Aortic stenosis	3
Abdominal or thoracic surgery	3
Patient in 'poor medical condition'	3

Patient's score	Incidence of death	Incidence of severe cardiovascular complications
≥26	56%	22%
6–25	4%	17%
≤5	0.2%	0.7%

It is extremely important to identify patients at risk of perioperative myocardial ischaemia, as MI in surgical patients carries 50% mortality, much higher than those presenting from the general population. Once identified, these patients can have their condition optimised if possible, appropriate arrangements can be made for anaesthesia and postoperative monitoring. It may even be wise to discuss with the patient if they wish to proceed with an operation if their risk seems disproportionately and inappropriately high.

Risk of perioperative re-infarction following a previous MI
0–3 months → 30%
3–6 months → 15%
>6 months → 6%
This may be significantly reduced with perioperative intensive care.

Recent research has suggested that the perioperative risk of MI is not as high as previously thought. The risk after a previous infarction is related less to the age of the infarction than to the functional status of the ventricles and the amount of myocardium at risk from further ischaemia.

New recommendations suggest the period within 6 weeks of infarction as a time of *high* risk for a perioperative cardiac event (6 weeks = mean healing time of the infarct related lesion). The period from 6 weeks to 3 months is of *intermediate* risk. In uncomplicated cases, there appears to be no benefit in delaying surgery more than 3 months after a MI. This is in contrast to the research of the 1980s.

The important questions to ask when seeing a patient are:

1. Is this patient at risk?

2. Can the patient's present treatment be improved?

All patients should be optimally treated prior to elective surgery. Any subsequent risk should be explained to them and an appropriate perioperative plan made with all concerned. Those at high risk substantially benefit from perioperative intensive care. The subsections below describe the management of different manifestations of cardiac disease. It is important to remember that it is only worth ordering investigations and tests (which sometimes carry their own morbidity and mortality and take time) if the result is likely to substantially alter patient management.

Ischaemic heart disease and angina

Chronic stable angina, in its own right, has a limited impact on risk. More important is functional history. The severity of angina can be estimated from the history. Patients who experience angina with minimal exertion, for example dressing, or at rest, are most at risk of perioperative MI.

Those reporting severe symptoms should be investigated with an exercise tolerance test if they are able to walk. Those who for any reason cannot walk, for example osteoarthritis or peripheral vascular disease of the lower limb, may undergo more sophisticated tests for myocardial ischaemia, such as dobutamine stress testing or thallium scanning to identify areas of myocardial ischaemia. Such patients may go on to have coronary angiography, angioplasty or even coronary artery bypass grafting. Otherwise it may be possible to optimise the angina with nitrates, calcium channel blockers or β-blockers. The extent of investigation depends on the extent of surgery and its urgency.

Unstable angina suggests acute myocardial ischaemia and should be controlled prior to surgery. In general all cardiovascular drugs should be continued right up to surgery. Patients 'nil by mouth' for elective surgery must continue to take all normal medication (with small sips of water if required).

Hypertension

Uncontrolled hypertension is associated with increased perioperative morbidity. The precise level of acceptability is controversial. Many anaesthetists will anaesthetise patients with hypertension up to 115 mmHg diastolic, however most will be concerned with any pressures above 200 mmHg systolic or 100 mmHg diastolic. To help exclude a stress effect, always record blood pressure at preassessment and take a history of previous control with measurements. These patients often benefit from anxiolytic premedication. Acute treatment of hypertension for elective surgery is contraindicated. Asymptomatic or 'Silent' myocardial ischaemia can occur in untreated hypertensives undergoing surgery, resulting in increased perioperative morbidity and mortality.

Cardiac failure

A history of cardiac failure is the single best predictor for poor outcome after surgery. Functional history, a chest X-ray and any recent echocardiogram will help quantify this. Reduced left ventricular function increases risk. It is essential to optimise the condition of any patient with cardiac failure, especially if it is decompensated or uncontrolled. Such patients will require admission to the Intensive Care Unit (ICU) for specialised invasive monitoring and are likely to require inotropic drugs if surgery cannot be postponed.

Information from echocardiography

- Valvular heart disease – diagnosis and severity
- Left ventricular function:
  - good/moderate/poor
- Wall movement abnormalities
- Chamber dilatation

Cardiac dysrhythmias

The presence of an arrhythmia implies that a patient has cardiac disease, which is likely to be ischaemic in origin. The Goldman cardiac risk index shows that patients with dysrhythmias are at increased risk of perioperative morbidity and mortality. It is therefore important to diagnose, investigate and treat patients who present for surgery with an arrhythmia. Occasionally an elderly patient may present with atrial fibrillation (AF) that has not been detected previously. Often the AF will be

1

well rate-controlled (ventricular rate <100/min) and is probably chronic. This may not need immediate treatment, but this depends on the type of surgery and the experience of the anaesthetist. Patients in AF with a ventricular response rate >100/min should be referred to the cardiologists or general physicians who will weigh up the relative risks and benefits of either controlling ventricular rate with drugs like digoxin, or attempting cardioversion back to sinus rhythm. The urgency and extent of surgery is also taken into account. However, all patients with AF should be considered for anticoagulation postoperatively, especially those who have left atrial hypertrophy documented by echocardiography.

The presence of heart block on the preoperative ECG can also affect outcome after surgery (Table 1.4). It was once thought that atrioventricular conduction delays worsened during anaesthesia and surgery, leading to a risk of complete, or third degree, heart block and catastrophic decline in cardiac output. Further investigation has left the situation less clear, and opinion is divided about how to treat patients presenting for surgery with bi- and trifascicular block. The table shows a likely approach that a typical anaesthetist might take, although there are always exceptions to the rule and it is wise to alert the anaesthetist to any patient with heart block.

Valvular heart disease

All patients with known valve dysfunction should have a recent echocardiogram (ideally <6 months) and all newly diagnosed murmurs should have an echocardiogram. Symptomatic valvular disease carries a very high risk with surgery. Syncope is a particularly worrying symptom. Such patients and those with severe disease may benefit from surgical correction prior to any other procedure. Regional anaesthesia can be particularly hazardous in patients unable to increase their cardiac output in response to a decreased systemic vascular resistance. Such patients often have critical stenotic valvular lesions. These patients require antibiotic prophylaxis to prevent infective endocarditis. Current indications and regimens can be found in the British National Formulary© and confirmed by local Microbiology departments.

Patients with prosthetic heart valves or heart valve defects will always require prophylactic antibiotics, whether the valve replacement is mechanical or tissue. Their heart sounds and murmurs may be difficult to interpret and an echocardiogram may be required to assess valve function. Attention will also need to be paid to anticoagulation (see Chapter 8: Perioperative management of coagulation).

Pacemakers

Diathermy during surgery and muscle fasciculations with suxamethonium (a short acting muscle relaxant) can interfere with some pacemakers.

Table 1.4 Summary of heart block

Type of heart block	Description	ECG appearance	Likely action
First degree heart block	P-R interval is >0.2 s	P QRS T P QRS T	■ None ■ Probably not clinically significant
Second degree heart block: ■ Mobitz type I (Wenckebach)	P-R interval lengthens with successive beats until a beat is dropped (no QRS complex)	PQRS T P QRS T P QRS T P P QRS T drop	■ Rarely proceeds to complete heart block ■ No action required
■ Mobitz type II	Block distal to the A-V node which may occur regularly, for example every 2nd or 3rd beat (2:1, 3:1 block respectively)	P QRS T P P QRS T P P QRS T 2:1 block	■ At risk of evolving into third degree, or complete heart block perioperatively ■ May need temporary cardiac pacing
Third degree heart block also known as complete heart block	No A-V conduction. Atria and ventricles beat independently. Ventricular rate likely to be low due to less frequent production of cardiac action potentials by ventricular muscle	P P P P P P P QRS T QRS T	■ Very high risk of cardiovascular collapse during or after surgery ■ Refer to cardiologist ■ Elective patients will require permanent pacing before surgery

1

Table 1.4 continued

Type of heart block	Description	ECG appearance	Likely action
			■ Temporary pacing can be established preoperatively in an urgent or emergency case or if there is sepsis
Right bundle branch block	QRS complex >0.12 s S wave in lead I, RSR pattern in lead V₁	P → QRS → T V₁	■ Common ■ Not usually significant, unless associated with left or right axis deviation which implies 'bifascicular' block ■ May lead to complete heart block in the elderly
Left bundle branch block	QRS complex >0.12 s wide R waves in leads I and V₄₋₆	P → QRS → T V₆	■ Implies significant cardiac disease
Partial trifascicular block	Bifascicular block plus first degree heart block	P → QRS → T V₁ Plus axis deviation	■ Particularly likely to progress to complete heart block ■ Pacing essential

This is particularly true of more sophisticated programmable models. Therefore it is important to know the precise type of pacemaker and the date of the last check. This should have been within 6 months. A good history is essential, as co-existing disease is common (50% have ischaemic heart disease, 20% are hypertensive and 10% are diabetic). A recurrence of symptoms (e.g. dizziness or syncope) may indicate pacemaker malfunction. Essential investigations include an ECG, CXR and electrolytes.

Conclusion

First identify and then optimise cardiovascular disease. Plan the required investigations well in advance as some may take time (e.g. echocardiogram) and liaise with senior anaesthetic staff early. It is clear that the risks of cardiovascular complications can be substantially reduced with sensible planning and appropriate perioperative care.

Key points

1. Cardiovascular disease is common amongst patients presenting for surgery.

2. Unstable or severe disease must be fully optimised prior to elective surgery.

3. Persistent hypertension needs treatment and rescheduling of elective surgery.

4. Do not forget infective endocarditis antibiotic prophylaxis for 'at-risk' cases.

Further reading

1 Chassot P-G, Delabays A and Spahn DR. Preoperative evaluation of patients with, or at risk of, coronary artery disease undergoing non-cardiac surgery. Br J Anaesth 2002; 89(5): 747–759.

2 Mangano DT, et al. Effect of atenolol on mortality and cardiovascular morbidity after non-cardiac surgery. NEJM 1996; 335: 1713–1720.

3 ACC/AHA Pocket Guideline Update. Perioperative Cardiovascular Evaluation for Non-cardiac Surgery. A Report of American College of Cardiology/American Heart Association Task Force on Practice Guidelines, November 2002.

2

Perioperative management of respiratory disease

Tim Clarke

2

Respiratory disease is common in patients presenting for surgery whatever their age. The disease can be acute, chronic or acute-on-chronic with a wide range of functional physiological deficit. The respiratory component can be the primary pathology (e.g. asthma) or secondary (e.g. heart failure presenting as asthma) or a restrictive defect (in severe ankylosing spondylitis).

Most of these patients requiring anaesthesia will be undergoing surgery unrelated to their respiratory problems but which is unlikely to improve lung function. Long periods of postoperative hypoxaemia can lead to myocardial and cerebral ischaemia or infarction. Careful planning with pre- and postoperative preparation and optimisation will significantly reduce morbidity.

Common diseases

Asthma
Characterised by reversible, small airway constriction leading to increased airway resistance. Can be classified as allergic, IgE mediated or non-allergic. Affects 7–10% children (males:females 2:1) and 3–5% adults (no sex difference beyond 30 years).

Chronic obstructive pulmonary disease (COPD)
Describes a range of conditions categorised as emphysema, chronic bronchitis and asthmatic bronchitis. There may be some reversible element to the bronchoconstriction.

Others
Patients suffering from less common but nevertheless important conditions should be made known to the anaesthetist. These include diseases such as obstructive sleep apnoea, Pickwickian syndrome (alveolar hypoventilation syndrome) and any patients on home oxygen or other breathing devices (e.g. nasal continuous positive airway pressure, CPAP).

History

- Current functional ability as compared to when at their best (including peak flow readings).
- Disease history, hospitalisations.
- Current treatment.
- Drug history and allergies. The patient may be taking steroids. Their perioperative management is described in Chapter 9: Perioperative management of steroid therapy.

- Current infection, sputum.

- Smoking.

- Previous anaesthesia, and any anaesthetic complications.

- Cardiac history. Respiratory and cardiac diseases often go hand in hand.

Examination and investigations

2

- Observation, e.g. short of breath at rest, respiratory rate, cyanosis, pursed lip breathing, use of accessory muscles, oxygen mask.

- Full systemic examination with emphasis on chest auscultation.

- Peak flow, pre and post bronchodilators.

- Spirometry/vitalograph, pre and post bronchodilators.

- Pulse oximetry – the long-standing hypoxaemia of a patient with chronic lung disease may result in a peripheral oxygen saturation (S_po_2) in the low 90 or even high 80 percents when breathing air. It is useful to have a baseline reading to know whether the patient's respiratory function is normal for them when deciding an appropriate amount of supplemental oxygen to prescribe, or when discontinuing oxygen therapy.

- Electrocardiogram (ECG) – may provide evidence of dysrhythmias (for example atrial fibrillation or flutter with acute pneumonia), right heart strain in cor pulmonale or acute pulmonary embolus (S wave in lead I, Q and inverted T waves in lead III, right axis deviation).

- Chest X-ray (CXR) – not essential for all patients; there are likely to be local guidelines in each hospital.

- Full blood count (FBC) may reveal evidence of polycythaemia or infection.

- Urea and electrolytes (U&Es) – possible hypokalaemia with β_2-agonists.

- Arterial blood gases – raised bicarbonate may indicate chronic CO_2 retention. When recording arterial blood gases, always remember to note down the concentration of oxygen that the patient was breathing at the time (air = 21% oxygen). Respiratory failure is defined as an arterial P_ao_2 of 8.0 kPa or less when breathing air. It is divided into type I and type II.

2

Type I respiratory failure	Type II respiratory failure
P_aO_2 <8.0 kPa on air	P_aO_2 <8.0 kPa on air
P_aCO_2 normal or low (normal range 4.5–6.0 kPa)	P_aCO_2 exceeds 6.5 kPa
Caused by failure of gas exchange across alveolar membrane to pulmonary capillaries	Caused by a reduction in alveolar ventilation due to a decrease in tidal volume

Examples:
■ Chest infection
■ Asthma
■ Pulmonary oedema
■ Pulmonary embolus
	Examples:
	■ Acute exacerbation of chronic obstructive pulmonary disease
	■ Non-respiratory:
	  • opioid analgesics
	  • head injury

	Notes: A subgroup of these patients may be sensitive to high concentrations of oxygen. Normally respiratory drive is controlled by chemoreceptors that detect rising P_aCO_2 and stimulate breathing. It is thought that some patients with chronically high P_aCO_2 lose this drive to breathe, and rely instead upon hypoxia, which normally plays little role. Thus high concentrations of supplemental oxygen may cause apnoea – although there is a body of opinion that does not believe this hypothesis

Pulmonary function tests (in average adult)

PFT	Normal	Emphysema	Bronchitis	Asthma
FVC	≥3–4 L	Decreased	Normal or slightly decreased	Decreased
FEV_1	>2–3 L	Decreased	Normal or slightly decreased	Decreased
TLC	5–7 L	Increased	Normal or slightly decreased	Decreased
RV	1–2 L	Increased	Increased	Increased

Hypoxaemia/ hypercarbia		Late in disease	Early in disease	Acute attack only
Diffusion capacity	Normal	Decreased	Normal or slightly decreased	Normal

FVC	Forced vital capacity
FEV$_1$	Forced expiratory volume in 1 second
TLC	Total lung capacity
RV	Residual volume

2

Preoperative optimisation

■ Ideally the patient should stop smoking. Nicotine is an adrenergic agonist which increases blood pressure, increases myocardial oxygen demand and may reduce coronary blood flow. Carbon monoxide in cigarette smoke combines avidly with haemoglobin to form carboxyhaemoglobin, which cannot carry oxygen. These effects are reduced after 12–24 h abstinence. Cigarette smoke also reduces ciliary and immunological function in the lungs that takes up to 2 months to recover.

■ Drug therapy; continue normal medications, medical consultation if inadequate.

■ Treat current infection.

■ Chest physiotherapy, continue postoperatively.

■ Postoperative analgesia plan.

■ Book HDU/ICU bed.

Anaesthesia

■ In patients with severe respiratory disease, is the operation really necessary? Do the risks of anaesthesia outweigh the benefits of surgery?

■ Local anaesthetic alternative. Regional anaesthesia is not risk free. Spinals and epidurals cause a fall in FRC and an interscalene brachial plexus block may block the phrenic nerve. However, postoperative analgesia is often excellent allowing coughing and physiotherapy. Often used in combination with general anaesthesia.

■ Premedication. Anxiolysis is important but should be used with caution as benzodiazepines cause respiratory centre depression. Bronchodilators may be useful at this time.

■ All volatile anaesthetic agents are bronchodilators.

Postoperative period

■ Administer supplemental oxygen, which should be humidified if possible to prevent secretions from desiccating. When administering oxygen to patients with type II respiratory failure it is wise to use a fixed performance facemask, i.e. one that delivers a fixed concentration of oxygen irrespective of the patient's breathing pattern. Major abdominal or thoracic surgery may precipitate or exacerbate type I respiratory failure. In this case, the concentration of oxygen is less important, and the oxygen can be delivered via a standard, variable performance mask. The efficacy of this treatment should be determined by monitoring S_pO_2, respiratory rate or even arterial blood gases. The concept of the P_aO_2/F_IO_2 ratio is useful when assessing a patient's progress on treatment or the effects of changing treatment (see Chapter 27: Perioperative scenarios).

■ Analgesia is paramount, especially after major chest or abdominal surgery. Patients that are unable to cough without substantial discomfort will not be able to clear mucous secretions in the lower airways. Soon the small airways become blocked and the alveoli beyond collapse ('base atelectasis'). As the alveoli are perfused by blood but not ventilated, they increase right-to-left shunt. This can only be resolved by re-expanding collapsed areas of lung with physiotherapy or CPAP, not simply by increasing F_IO_2. Base atelectasis also predisposes to the development of pneumonia.

■ Restart regular medication promptly.

■ Regular physiotherapy.

■ Postoperative ventilation. Consider each patient individually. Rough guidelines – if FEV_1 <1L, FVC <70% (of predicted) or FEV_1/FVC <50% (of predicted), the patient may require ventilation in the postoperative period.

Key points

1. Respiratory disease affects patients of all ages.

2. Patients should be near to their functional 'best' prior to anaesthesia and surgery, if possible.

3. The majority of problems will be in the postoperative period.

4. Accurate and thorough preoperative assessment and patient education can limit morbidity postoperatively.

Further reading

Nunn JF et al. Respiratory criteria of fitness for surgery and anaesthesia. Anaesthesia 1988; 43(7): 543–551.

3

Perioperative care of children

Warren Fisher

Introduction

Children present a range of problems for their carers. They present in a range of ages, a range of sizes and with a range of clinical conditions greatly different from adults. They are prone to unpredictability, sometimes temperamental, often scared by the environment of healthcare and come with parents or guardians who need just as much support as the child. There are significant anatomical, physiological, pharmacodynamic and pharmacokinetic differences between adults and children. In short, when you care for a child you deal with a whole different entity.

This chapter is designed to highlight some of the issues and provide some practical help in the perioperative care of children for surgery.

Preoperative preparation

■ Assessment

■ Special circumstances

■ Premedication

Assessment

Assessment of children for surgery follows traditional lines of History, Examination and Investigation, but there are features of the history which will be of particular interest.

■ History: asthma, bronchitis, prematurity (+/− neonatal ventilation), heart problems, epilepsy, other medical conditions

■ Cardiorespiratory function: is the child well at present, recent coughs and colds, wheezing, exercise tolerance, dyspnoea with feeds for infants/babies

■ Feeding, vomiting, weight gain, including timing of last feed/drink

■ Previous surgery and anaesthesia (any problems or family problems with anaesthesia?)

■ Medications and allergies

■ Loose teeth

Subsequent examination of a child will be guided by the history. It will often be an opportunistic approach to examination which will depend on establishing a rapport with the child and on the participation of the parent.

The history and examination should guide investigations in children and while there may be little place for the routine blood tests that are taken in adults, appropriate investigations are mandatory where there is a good indication. In some cases, where blood sampling is known to be difficult, it is worthwhile discussing the investigations with senior clinicians. It may be possible to delay tests until the child is anaesthetised, which may save the veins as well as a great deal of stress to child and clinician alike. A bad experience will affect ongoing care!

Major investigations such as CT or MRI scans will need careful planning, since many children will require some form of sedation for such procedures.

Common problems

Coughs and colds

A large number of children who present for surgery, particularly during the winter months, will have a current or recent respiratory tract infection (RTI). There is evidence to suggest that children with a current infection are at increased risk during anaesthesia and may be particularly prone to laryngospasm and episodes of desaturation. The period of risk may extend to as long as 6 weeks after an infection. If no child were anaesthetised during this time period there would clearly be some children who would never be suitable for elective surgery.

A pragmatic compromise would be that the following patients are unsuitable for elective surgery:

- Very recent onset RTI
- Unwell child (parent may be the best judge)
- Pyrexia
- Lower respiratory tract signs on examination
- Underlying respiratory disease
- Infant with RTI

If there is doubt, early discussion with the anaesthetist is advisable.

Asthma

Many children have asthma or other chronic medical conditions. In general the condition should be assessed and optimised prior to surgery. In the case of asthma this may involve premedication with a β_2 agonist. Children with a respiratory tract infection should probably be delayed if possible and there are a small number of children with asthma in whom non-steroidal anti-inflammatory drugs (NSAIDs) should be avoided.

Heart murmurs

Most murmurs in children are innocent but a small proportion will indicate the presence of an underlying significant cardiac lesion and need investigation before surgery. Children with an abnormal heart may develop cardiac compromise during anaesthesia, will require antibiotic prophylaxis and may have associated significant abnormalities as part of a complex syndrome. Investigation is important.

Innocent murmurs are usually soft mid-systolic, with normal first and second heart sounds and are not associated with cardiac signs and symptoms.

Pathological murmurs may be associated with cardiac signs and symptoms, for example cyanosis. The murmur may be diastolic and/or systolic obscuring the heart sounds. It is likely to be loud and may be continuous.

If in doubt seek advice.

Premedication
Local anaesthetic creams (EMLA® or Ametop®)
■ Provide topical anaesthesia for venous cannulation

■ Require >1 h to work (amethocaine based take 45 min)

■ Need to be applied in the right place! (which may need to be marked before application)

■ Not needed if inhalational induction is planned (see below)

Sedatives
■ Benzodiazepines and opioids are commonly used

■ Provide anxiolysis

■ May help to improve co-operation at induction of anaesthesia

■ Need to be given at the right time (too early → worn off, too late → ineffective)

■ Most are oral preparations

Other premedication aims:
■ Drying of secretions

■ Prevention of bradycardia at induction

■ Acid aspiration prophylaxis

■ Analgesia

■ Continuation of long term medication

Preoperative fasting prior to surgery
■ Food/milk   6 h

■ Breast milk   4 h

■ Clear fluids   2–3 h

(clear fluids are clear enough to see through the full glass)

Induction of anaesthesia

■ To avoid the distress caused by venous cannulation, inhalational induction with sweet smelling agents (e.g. sevoflurane, halothane) is more frequently employed in children.

Postoperative care of children

Fluid management

The correct fluid management for individual cases clearly depends on the type of surgery performed and the medical requirements of the child. Rapid re-introduction of food and drink after surgery (particularly some reward foods such as burger and chips with cola or sweets even after minor surgery) will result in unpleasant consequences for children, parents and carpets alike. Gradual re-introduction of fluid followed by food is probably the wise approach.

For patients being kept off enteral feeds after an operation, there are many issues surrounding the type of fluid, the additives and the volume to be infused in any given time period. There are many different views on the type of fluid that should be given and there may be severe consequences if a child suffers from an error in prescribing (resulting in fluid overload or electrolyte imbalance).

Infants (children <1 year of age) and particularly those in the neonatal period (<44 weeks postconceptual age) may be at risk from hypoglycaemia. Any fluid regime must include an appropriate sugar content with monitoring of blood sugar levels.

A simple guide to volume of fluid to be infused in the older child above 6 months of age is the following:

Weight	Hourly fluid requirement
Up to 10 kg	4 ml/kg/h
10 to 20 kg	40 ml/h + 2 ml/h for each kg between 10 and 20 kg
>20 kg	40 ml/h + 20 ml/h + 1 ml/h for each kg above 20 kg

Fluid requirement calculations must also take into consideration abnormal losses such as:

■ Gastrointestinal: vomiting/nasogastric loss, diarrhoea, sequestration into gut

■ Increased insensible losses as a result of pyrexia or exposure

■ Bleeding

■ Preexisting deficit, e.g. prolonged fasting, preoperative dehydration

23

Postoperative analgesia

Analgesia in the perioperative period is a very complex subject and can involve complicated analgesic regimes after major surgery. However, the principles are simple and amenable to reason.

The main modalities of analgesia in current use are:

■ Simple analgesia, e.g. paracetamol, NSAIDs

■ Opioids, e.g. morphine, pethidine

■ Local anaesthetics, e.g. bupivacaine, lignocaine (lidocaine)

Each of the different classes of drugs may be administered in a wide variety of preparations, routes and timing schedules, such that even for the simple analgesic paracetamol, there is much debate about appropriate dosage regimes.

Opioids may be used in many different ways and when used in combination with local anaesthetics exhibit synergy (e.g. fentanyl used in combination with bupivacaine in epidural infusion). The combination may allow for a lower total mass of drug to be used and possibly reduce the side effects compared to the use of a single agent.

Local anaesthetics are used extensively in paediatric anaesthetic practice. Routes of administration include topical, infiltration, peripheral nerve block, plexus block and central block (spinal, caudal, epidural).

Any analgesic technique should balance the risks against the benefits. Individual drug dosages are beyond the scope of this chapter and the reader should refer to standard formularies for children.

Key points

1. Children are not merely scaled down adults.

2. They require different systems of care.

3. These are ideally separate from equivalent adult care.

4. Expertise and knowledge not just of the medicine of children, but also the care of children is essential to practice.

Further reading

Royal College of Paediatrics & Child Health, Paediatric Formulary.
Sumner E and Hatch DJ (Eds), Paediatric Anaesthesia, 2nd edn, Arnold 1999.

4

Perioperative management of the obese patient

Anand Sardesai

The number of obese patients presenting for surgery is increasing; the prevalence is increasing in the general population (15–20% and rising). Obese patients are more likely to suffer from comorbid disease and provide the anaesthetist with considerable challenges.

Definitions

Ideal body weight in kilograms (kg) = height (in cm) − [(100 for men) or (105 for women)].

Another measure commonly used clinically is:

$$\text{Body Mass Index (BMI)} = \text{Mass (in kg)}/[\text{height (in m)}]^2$$

A BMI of		
	$<25 \, kg/m^2$	= Normal
	$25\text{–}30 \, kg/m^2$	= Overweight
	$>30 \, kg/m^2$	= Obese
	$>35 \, kg/m^2$	= Morbidly obese
	$>55 \, kg/m^2$	= Super-morbidly obese

There is an increase in incidence of morbidity and mortality in patients with BMI $>30 \, kg/m^2$.

Obesity causes pathophysiological changes in all body systems, many of which are relevant in the perioperative period.

Cardiovascular system

There is an increase in the total blood volume but the volume to weight ratio is reduced. Blood volume is 50 ml/kg in obese patients compared to 75 ml/kg in non-obese individuals. Due to increases in metabolic demands there is an increase in stroke volume and cardiac output. This results in hypertrophy and dilatation of the left ventricle leading to diastolic dysfunction initially and systolic dysfunction later. Due to associated sleep apnoea and obesity hypoventilation syndrome, there is an increased incidence of hypoxia and hypoventilation. This causes hypoxic pulmonary vasoconstriction and pulmonary hypertension, which can lead to right heart failure.

There is an increased risk of arrhythmias secondary to ventricular hypertrophy, hypoxaemia, fatty infiltration of the cardiac conduction system, coronary artery disease and increased catecholamines. The incidence of ischaemic heart disease is greater due to associated hypertension, diabetes mellitus, hypercholesterolaemia and atherosclerosis.

There is a direct relationship between the prevalence of cardiovascular disease and BMI.

BMI	Prevalence of cardiovascular disease
<25 kg/m²	10%
25–30 kg/m²	21%
>30 kg/m²	37%

Respiratory system

Oxygen consumption and carbon dioxide production are increased in the obese as a result of metabolic activity of the excess fat and the increased workload on supportive tissues. Normocapnoea is maintained by hyperventilation at the cost of further increasing oxygen consumption. If inadequate oxygen is delivered to meet this demand, hypoxaemia occurs. Respiratory function will further decline leading to a vicious cycle of falling P_aO_2.

Increasing BMI is associated with an exponential decline in respiratory compliance. This decrease in compliance is a combination of a decrease in chest wall compliance due to fat deposition and a decrease in lung compliance due to an increase in blood volume. A decrease in compliance is associated with a decrease in functional residual capacity (FRC) and impairment of gas exchange. Some airways at the lung bases are almost always in a state of collapse, so alveoli are not ventilated. However, they are still perfused with blood causing an increased shunt. There is also an increase in airway resistance. These physiological changes result in a shallow and rapid breathing pattern which itself requires more energy and oxygen to sustain. Apart from a reduction in FRC there is a reduction in expiratory reserve volume and total lung capacity. Obesity is associated with obstructive sleep apnoea (OSA) in 5% of morbidly obese patients. A long-term consequence of OSA is the occurrence of central apnoeic events that ultimately lead to type II respiratory failure, pulmonary hypertension and right heart failure.

Gastrointestinal system

There is an increased risk of aspiration of gastric contents at induction of anaesthesia due to increased intra-abdominal pressure, increased volume of gastric contents and an increased incidence of hiatus hernia.

Pharmacokinetics

Absorption of drugs by the oral route is the same as other patients, however serum levels of drugs administered by other routes can be substantially

4

altered by increases in fat, body mass, cardiac output and blood volume. Increased fat stores increase the volume of distribution of many drugs and may increase requirements for, and clearance time of, fat soluble anaesthetics such as thiopentone. There may be variable effects of obesity on protein binding of drugs. The increased concentration of triglycerides, lipoproteins, cholesterol and free fatty acids may inhibit protein binding of some drugs, increasing their concentration.

Renal clearance of drugs increases due to increased renal blood flow and glomerular filtration rate.

This combination of factors means that recommended doses of drugs may have unpredictable effects in the obese.

Preoperative assessment

A history and full clinical examination are mandatory to exclude obesity-associated diseases such as:

Cardiovascular	Hypertension, ischaemic heart disease, cerebrovascular and peripheral vascular disease, deep venous thrombosis
Respiratory	Obstructive sleep apnoea, obesity hypoventilation syndrome
Endocrine	Diabetes mellitus, Cushing's syndrome
Gastrointestinal	Hiatus hernia, gallstones

Airway management in the obese may be particularly challenging due to fat face and cheeks, large breasts and an increase in soft tissues in the perioral area which may make intubation difficult. It may be necessary to do an awake fibreoptic intubation.

Locating a peripheral vein in which to place an adequately-sized cannula may also be very challenging.

It may be necessary to book a bed in a high dependency unit for postoperative observation of the patient.

Preoperative investigations

- Weight and height should be formally measured, not estimated, and recorded in metric units, to allow calculation of BMI

- Full blood count

- Urea and electrolytes

- Liver function tests. Liver function may be diminished by fatty infiltration

■ Electrocardiogram for evidence of myocardial ischaemia or right heart failure

■ Blood glucose – to detect type II diabetes mellitus

■ Chest X-ray

The anaesthetist should be consulted preoperatively, as additional investigations might be needed. The operating theatres should be contacted as additional personnel and equipment may be required to move the patient during and after anaesthesia.

Premedication

All morbidly obese patients should receive prophylaxis against acid aspiration. A combination of a H_2 blocker (e.g. ranitidine 150 mg orally) and a drug to increase gastric emptying (e.g. metoclopramide 10 mg orally) given 12 h and 2 h before surgery will reduce the risk of aspiration of acid stomach contents. 30 ml of 0.3 M sodium citrate (a non-particulate antacid) can be given immediately before induction.

Most of the patient's medications including cardiovascular drugs and steroids should be continued as normal until the time of surgery, although it is recommended that angiotensin converting enzyme inhibitors be stopped on the day before surgery, as their continuation can lead to profound hypotension during anaesthesia.

In a diabetic patient blood glucose levels should be monitored perioperatively and if necessary a sliding scale should be started (see Chapter 11: Perioperative management of diabetes).

Prophylactic measures to prevent deep vein thrombosis should be used and continued into the postoperative phase until the patient is fully mobile (e.g. compression stocking and low dose subcutaneous heparin).

Obese patients are at increased risk of developing wound infection and may require prophylactic antibiotics.

4

Intraoperative management

Positioning
Most operating tables are designed for patients weighing up to 120–140 kg. The combination of two operating tables may be required for the obese patient.

Regional anaesthesia

Use of regional anaesthesia in the obese reduces the risks of difficult intubation and acid aspiration and also provides safer and more effective postoperative analgesia. Regional anaesthesia in the obese can be technically challenging due to difficulties identifying the usual anatomical landmarks.

Postoperative period

Postoperative morbidity and mortality in the obese patient is increased compared to the non-obese patient. Wound infection is twice as common. The likelihood of deep vein thrombosis and the risk of pulmonary embolism are increased, emphasising the importance of early postoperative ambulation. Pulmonary complications are frequent, especially after abdominal surgery. The semi-sitting position is often used during the postoperative period in an attempt to decrease the likelihood of arterial hypoxaemia. Arterial oxygenation should be closely monitored and supplemental oxygen provided as indicated by pulse oximetry or the P_aO_2 (partial pressure of oxygen in blood). The maximum decrease in P_aO_2 typically occurs 2 to 3 days postoperatively. Measures to avoid pulmonary complications due to the development of base atelectasis include nursing the patient in a semi-recumbent position (30–45 degrees), use of humidified gases and early chest physiotherapy. Nocturnal use of nasal continuous positive airway pressure (CPAP) can be useful in the presence of obstructive sleep apnoea. Good postoperative analgesia is essential, as is early mobilisation to reduce postoperative complications.

Patient controlled analgesia (PCA) – with opioid drugs can provide good pain relief and the dose should be based on ideal body weight. Supplemental oxygen, close observation and pulse oximetry monitoring are recommended.

Epidural opioids are preferred to the intravenous route, allowing administration of a smaller dose resulting in less sedation and fewer respiratory complications.

Obese patients in the intensive care unit

Obese patients are more likely to develop respiratory complications. The tidal volume set on the ventilator should be based on the patient's lean body weight in order to reduce the incidence of barotrauma. Positive end expiratory pressure may help to prevent airway collapse. Elective tracheostomy may be helpful in weaning the patient from the ventilator.

Invasive haemodynamic monitoring is helpful in titrating fluid replacement and assessing cardiac performance. Siting of central venous catheters may be difficult.

Key points

1. Obesity affects multiple systems in the body.

2. A thorough understanding of pathophysiology and specific complications is essential in order to manage obese patients.

3. Thorough preoperative assessment of the obese patient is mandatory, to identify and optimise any comorbid conditions.

4. It is advisable to discuss pre- and postoperative management of morbidly obese patients with the anaesthetist.

Further reading
Adams JP and Murphy PG. Obesity in anaesthesia and intensive care. Br J Anaesth 2000; 85:91–108.

4

5

Perioperative management of the elderly patient

Karen Pedersen

Introduction

Ageing is a continuum rather than an abrupt event. However, it is customary to consider the geriatric population to be persons aged 65 years and older. This group currently comprises about 15% of the Western population and one quarter of all surgical patients and will increase in size as life expectancy increases. The cost of caring for this growing population will rise steadily. This is not only due to increasing numbers but also to the advent and uptake of new diagnostic and therapeutic technologies and drugs.

Life expectancy is a measure of typical longevity and is currently moving into the 9th decade.

The geriatric population is not only subject to the changes caused by ageing. Age-related diseases also affect them.

Ageing can be defined as a progressive, universally prevalent physiological process that produces measurable changes in the structure and function of tissues and organs. However, there are marked differences between individuals in their maximal capacity at somatic maturity (about 30 years of age) and in the rate at which decline occurs. This is borne out by the observation that some elderly people appear much 'younger' than others of the same chronological age. The mechanism of ageing has not been fully elucidated but is probably related to a decrease in cellular energy production due to deterioration of the mitochondrial genome.

Changes due to age related diseases are not present in all elderly people and do not increase in severity in proportion to chronological age.

Physiology of ageing

The discussion that follows refers to changes due to age rather than those due to age related diseases. Such diseases must be identified and their physiological consequences assessed separately from changes due purely to ageing.

In general terms there is a 1% decline per year in the functional reserve of all organ systems.

Cardiovascular system

Changes

- decreased number and increased size of cardiac myocytes

- increased myocardial fibrosis and valvular calcification

- increased ventricular wall thickness

- decreased ventricular compliance

- increased large artery stiffness

- reduced maximal cardiac output (about 1% per year)

■ reduced maximal heart rate

■ increased time required for myocardial contraction and relaxation

■ blunted beta-adrenoceptor mediated contractile and inotropic responses

Implications

■ cardiac output is volume dependent and yet the heart is volume intolerant

■ greater dependence on the atrial contribution to late diastolic filling leading to severe compromise of cardiac output with the loss of sinus rhythm

Respiratory system

Changes

■ deterioration of lung elastin leading to increased lung compliance and decreased lung recoil

■ decreased total alveolar surface area due to breakdown of alveolar septa

■ increased alveolar and anatomical dead space

■ increased residual volume at the expense of expiratory reserve volume

■ increased functional residual capacity (FRC) at the expense of vital capacity (VC)

■ increased closing volume and closing capacity to exceed FRC leading to small airway closure even during normal tidal ventilation

■ increased ventilation-perfusion mismatching

■ decreased chest wall compliance due to fibrosis and calcification

Implications

■ increased work of breathing and limited maximal breathing capacity

■ impaired oxygenation with increased alveolar-arterial oxygen gradient

■ decreased efficiency of carbon dioxide elimination

■ decreased ventilatory response to hypoxia and hypercarbia should they develop before or after surgery. Opioid analgesics are common culprits

Central nervous system

Changes

■ decreased brain mass due to loss of neurons

■ proportionate decrease in total brain blood flow

5

- depletion of neurotransmitters such as dopamine, norepinephrine and serotonin

- increased activity of catabolic enzymes such as monoamine oxidase and catechol O-methyltransferase

- decreased CNS plasticity and ability to recover from injury

- language skills, personality, information comprehension and long-term memory well maintained

- short-term memory impaired and visual and auditory reaction times slowed

Implications

- decreased ability to recover from injury such as stroke

- decreased anaesthetic requirements

- there is no reason to assume that the elderly surgical patient does not meet legal standards for mental competence

Peripheral nervous system and neuromuscular function

Changes

- progressive deafferentation of both sensory and motor pathways

- decreased dynamic muscle strength and control

Implications

- increased threshold for virtually all forms of perception

Autonomic nervous system

Changes

- deafferentation of neurones in the sympathoadrenal pathways

- decreased adrenal mass (15% less by age 80)

- increased plasma levels of norepinephrine

- decreased number of receptors

- decreased affinity for agonist molecules

- impairment of adenylate cyclase activation

Implications

- 'beta-blockade of ageing' with marked decrease in end organ responsiveness, e.g. blunted cardiac inotropic and chronotropic responses to stimulation by beta agonists

Renal system

Changes

- decreased mass of kidneys

- decreased number of functional units

- decreased total renal blood flow (medulla mostly spared)

- glomerular sclerosis

- glomerular filtration rate (GFR) decreases more than renal plasma flow due to compensatory increases in filtration fraction

Body composition and metabolism

Changes

- increased lipid fraction

- loss of skeletal muscle

- glucose intolerance

- decreased maximal oxygen consumption

- decreased basal metabolic activity

- plasma volume well maintained in the healthy elderly population

- decreased serum albumin and decreased protein binding

Implications

- increased reservoir for anaesthetics and other lipid soluble drugs

- decreased production of heat and decreased ability to maintain core temperature despite normal hypothalamic thermostatic set points

Haematological and immune systems

Changes

- decreased total bone marrow mass

- decreased spleen size

- increased erythrocyte fragility (not enough to decrease erythrocyte life span in vivo)

Implications

- clinically significant anaemia or coagulopathy always due to pathology but there is a decreased response to imposed anaemia

- decreased immune competence

5

Drugs

Both pharmacokinetics and pharmacodynamics are altered in the elderly.

Pharmacokinetics

■ drug distribution is affected by a decrease in total body water and lean body mass, relative increase in body fat (may lead to an increased volume of distribution of fat soluble drugs), decreased serum albumin (may lead to increased free portion of drugs that are normally highly protein bound), increased alpha 1 acid glycoprotein and a decreased cardiac output

■ hepatic metabolism and renal excretion are affected by age related changes in hepatic mass, hepatic and renal blood flow, hepatic enzyme activity, glomerular filtration rate and urine concentrating ability

The effect of ageing on analgesic requirements is not very well defined. Assessment of pain is confused by the fact that elderly people tend to be more stoical, less likely to report that they are in pain and less likely to request pain relief. However, a strong inverse relationship has been found between morphine and fentanyl patient controlled analgesia use and advancing age.

Elderly patients are often taking large numbers of medications that may interact with one another or with other drugs administered perioperatively. Due to a decrease in the functional reserve of all organ systems with advancing age and an increased prevalence of coexisting diseases, the elderly are much more likely to experience side effects. This is particularly true of cardiovascular drugs (e.g. hypotension and bradycardia with calcium channel blockers).

Preoperative assessment

Preoperative assessment of the elderly, as with any other patient presenting for surgery, includes weighing up the relative risks and benefits of the proposed procedure for the particular patient. This includes a thorough assessment of the patient's medical condition (including disease severity, stability and prior treatment), appropriate investigations, the institution of any necessary therapy to optimise the situation and obtaining informed consent.

Advanced age is not in itself a contraindication to surgery, although age over 75 years has been found to be associated with a high early mortality. The presence and severity of any co-morbidities is probably more important than the age of the patient *per se*.

Preoperative risk stratification is important as it makes very little sense to subject any patient to an operation if the perioperative morbidity and mortality are prohibitive. This can be done by considering the functional status of the patient, the presence of clinical predictors of increased perioperative risk and the surgery-specific risk of the proposed procedure.

A careful assessment of intravascular volume status and electrolyte balance should be made in all patients, particularly during non-elective surgery. Due to decreased functional reserve, any abnormalities present have far greater physiological implications than in younger patients and should be corrected prior to induction of anaesthesia if at all possible. Patients may be hypovolaemic due to dehydration, blood loss, sepsis and bowel preparation. Hypervolaemia may result from congestive cardiac failure or renal failure. Hypokalaemia may result from chronic diuretic treatment, vomiting or bowel preparation. The administration of hypo-osmolar replacement fluids on the ward may render patients hyponatraemic.

Poor preoperative preparation will increase the incidence of intra- and postoperative complications.

There is increasing evidence that the maintenance or initiation of beta blockade in the perioperative period in elderly patients at risk of or with ischaemic heart disease leads to decreased cardiac morbidity and mortality. This should be considered in all patients without contraindications.

A thorough evaluation of the mental status and competence of the elderly patient must be performed. Most elderly patients will meet the legal definition of mental competence. Informed consent must therefore be obtained. Any questions or concerns that the patient raises must be taken seriously. Paternalistic behaviour on the part of the physician must not be allowed to interfere with the patient's right to participate in decisions about their care.

5

Postoperative care

Common problems encountered postoperatively include hypo/hypertension, delayed wakening, pain, myocardial ischaemia, nausea and vomiting, agitation, oliguria, hypoxaemia, hypercarbia, laryngeal spasm and hypothermia. Most of these are both more common and more difficult to manage in the elderly. An important underlying principle of management is to determine the cause of the problem and then institute appropriate therapy as soon as possible. For example, hypertension due to the pain of a full bladder is best treated by an indwelling urinary catheter and not by vasoactive drugs or opioids.

Common causes for hypertension and hypotension in the postoperative period are:

Hypertension

Causes
■ preexisting hypertension

■ acute withdrawal of antihypertensive drugs, e.g. beta blockers

- pain

- hypercarbia

- hypoxia

- hypothermia

- myocardial infarction

- full bladder

- increased intracranial pressure

- surgical, e.g. carotid sinus denervation during neck dissection or carotid endarterectomy

Hypotension

Causes

- reduced preload (decreased venous return to the heart)
  - hypovolaemia (common)
  - vasodilatation (regional anaesthesia, drugs)
  - anaphylaxis
  - sepsis
  - increased abdominal pressure (intra-abdominal mass, ascites, distended bowel)
- reduced afterload (decreased systemic vascular resistance)
  - vasodilatation (regional anaesthesia, drugs)
  - severe acidosis
  - anaphylaxis
  - sepsis
- intrinsic cardiac problems
  - arrhythmias (particularly loss of atrial kick with atrial fibrillation causing reduced ventricular filling)
  - ischaemia
  - decreased myocardial contractility (age, acute myocardial infarction, residual anaesthetic drug effect)
  - valvular heart disease

Postoperative care does not cease once the patient leaves the recovery suite. They will require continual reassessment and treatment to avoid, identify and manage the broad range of problems elderly patients may encounter.

5

Key points

1. The elderly are a select group who present particular challenges in the perioperative period.

2. The elderly have less physiological reserve and tolerate acute pathophysiological change poorly.

3. Polypharmacy and altered pharmacokinetics and pharmacodynamics are significant problems in the elderly.

4. Careful preparation, patient selection and meticulous attention to detail, results in a successful outcome for the majority of these patients.

Further reading
1 Miller RD (ed.). Anaesthesia, 5th edn. Churchill Livingstone. 2000; 2140–2156.
2 Dodds C and Murray D. Preoperative assessment of the elderly. BJA CEPD Rev 2001; 1:181–184.

5

6

Perioperative management of emergency surgery

Jeremy Lermitte and Jonathan Hudsmith

Patients for emergency surgery present the anaesthetist with a number of challenging problems including an uncertain diagnosis, concomitant poorly-controlled medical conditions, a full stomach, dehydration, haemorrhage, pain and hypothermia. Thorough assessment is crucial as it allows the patient's condition to be optimised, the timing and technique of the anaesthetic to be ascertained and any potential problems to be preempted.

The approach to these patients can be divided into three phases:

■ preoperative

■ perioperative

■ postoperative

Preoperative phase

Visiting the patient allows an anaesthetic history to be taken and rapport to be established. Informed consent and explanation of procedures can be discussed and premedication (if indicated) can be prescribed. Particular emphasis is placed on the following factors:

Fluid status
Normal volumes

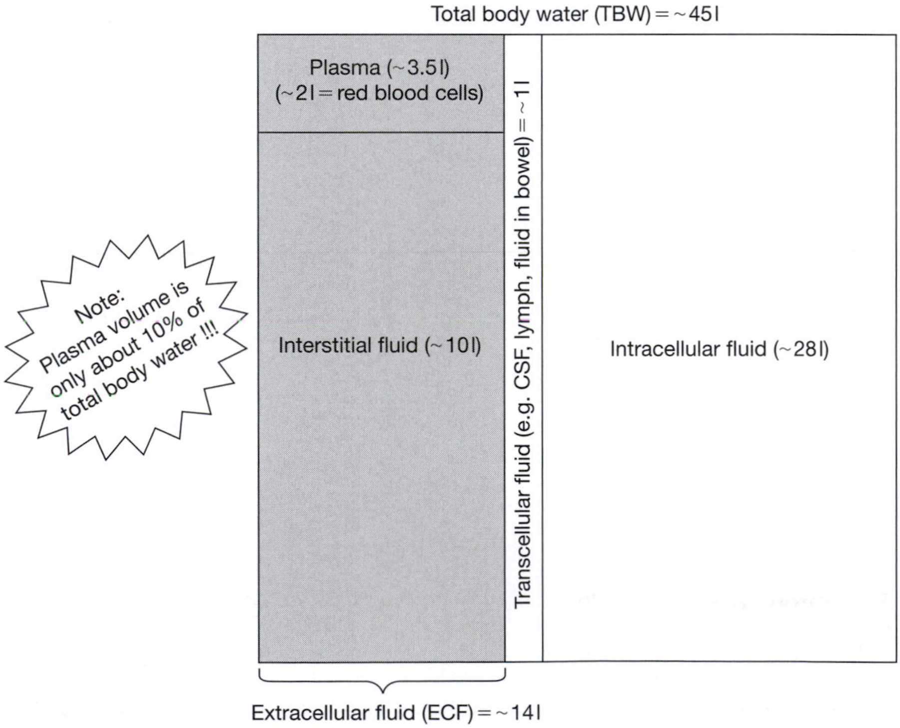

Note: Plasma volume is only about 10% of total body water !!!

Fig. 6.1 Typical distribution of fluid in a 70 kg adult male.

The '20 – 40 – 60' rule can be used to calculate the volumes in litres of extracellular, intracellular and total body water respectively of an adult (each number represents percentage of body weight). The extracellular volume of a 70 kg adult is 14 litres (20% of 70 kg). This volume can be further subdivided into the interstitial (15%) and plasma volume (5%). Blood volume is however greater than the plasma volume, due to the volume of the red blood cells and totals 7% body weight (70 ml/kg in the adult). Neonates have a high blood volume (80–90 ml/kg) and have higher total body water as a percentage of body weight (80%). The elderly and females have slightly lower amounts of body water (on average), due to increased fat which contains little water.

Deficits

Deficit of intravascular volume activates homeostatic mechanisms to maintain organ perfusion and oxygenation, by means of the renin-angiotensin-aldosterone system and release of steroid hormones from the adrenal cortex and catecholamines from the adrenal medulla. The combined action of these responses is to increase heart rate and force of contraction, cause arterial, arteriolar and venous vasoconstriction, increase respiratory rate and tidal volume, and increase water absorption in the loop of Henlé and distal convoluted tubule of the kidney. As losses become more substantial, these mechanisms are unable to maintain blood pressure. Those with good physiological reserve will be able to maintain blood pressure longer than those without. For example, a child's response to intravascular volume depletion will be to develop tachycardia. Blood pressure will only begin to fall with very severe fluid loss, and is a sign of impending cardiac arrest. Adults, and especially the elderly, will develop hypotension with less extreme losses (see Table 6.1).

Table 6.1 Intravascular deficits based on 70 kg adult

Class	1	2	3	4
Blood volume lost (%)	<15	15–30	30–40	>40
Heart rate	<100	>100	>120	>140
Blood pressure	Normal	Decreased pulse pressure	Decreased	Decreased
Respiratory rate	<20	20–30	30–40	>35
Urine output (ml/h)	>30	20–30	5–15	Small
Mental status	Normal	Anxious	Anxious/ confused	Confused/ lethargic

6

SHOCK = inadequate tissue perfusion to maintain that tissue's metabolic requirements

Causes of shock	Examples
Hypovolaemic	Haemorrhage, burns, dehydration
Cardiogenic	Left ventricular failure, myocardial infarction
Septic	Release of inflammatory molecules like cytokines, nitric oxide, platelet activating factor and products of the arachidonic acid pathway, which cause vasodilatation
Anaphylactic	Release of histamine in response to an antigen causes vasodilatation
Neurogenic	Spinal cord injury interrupts sympathetic autonomic nerve supply to vessels which normally maintain vasomotor tone
Adrenocortical insufficiency	Decreased plasma cortisol and ACTH levels result in loss of vasoconstrictor tone

Shock associated with intravascular deficits (blood loss) must first be distinguished from that of other origins. The degree of blood loss can then be ascertained and rectified (see Table 6.1). Interpretation of the table must consider age, athletic training, medications, hypothermia and pacemakers. Blood transfusions are associated with a number of risks including infection, electrolyte abnormalities and hypothermia (see Chapter 13: Transfusion and blood products). A haemoglobin of 8 g/dl is generally well tolerated by most patients, however this level may be tolerated poorly by the elderly and those with cardiorespiratory disease. In view of these considerations, blood loss up to 30% can be treated by fluid replacement with crystalloids or colloids alone. However, symptomatic patients and those with anticipated future losses should be transfused with blood.

Extracellular fluid deficits are difficult to detect in the early stages. Consideration must be given to the duration of the presenting condition and its pathophysiology. The extent of loss can be graded (see Table 6.2).

If fluid losses are isotonic only or long-standing the extracellular space is depleted. If hypotonic fluid is lost, there will be redistribution of fluid from the intracellular space. However any rehydration strategy should also aim to replenish fluid lost from the extracellular fluid (ECF) and intracellular fluid (ICF), especially since plasma volume is only about 10% of total body water (TBW).

Which replacement fluid?
This depends on which body fluid compartment is depleted. Blood, albumin and synthetic colloids largely remain in the intravascular space.

6

Table 6.2 **Extracellular deficits**

% body weight lost as water	Effect
<5	Thirst, dry membranes
5–10	Oliguria, orthostatic hypotension, sunken eyes, decreased skin turgor
>10	Shock, profound oliguria

Isotonic sodium containing fluids distribute to the extracellular space (25% of which is plasma). 5% glucose, which is hypotonic, distributes to all compartments and glucose saline distribution is dependent upon the ratio of saline to dextrose.

Why?

Sodium containing fluids distribute to the ECF only. Sodium ions (Na^+) are prevented from entering the ICF by the Na^+/K^+/ATPase pump. During infusion of 0.9% NaCl (normal saline), all the Na^+ remains in the ECF. 0.9% NaCl is isotonic and therefore there is no change in the osmolality of the ECF and no exchange of water across the cell membrane. 0.9% NaCl expands the ECF only. During infusion of 0.45% NaCl ('half-strength normal saline'), the osmolality of the ECF decreases, causing a shift of water from the ECF to the ICF. During infusion of 1.8% NaCl ('double-strength normal saline') the osmolality of the ECF increases, drawing water in from the ICF to maintain the osmotic balance.

Whilst infusions containing sodium expand the ECF, infusions of water (without sodium) expand the TBW. During infusion of 5% glucose, the glucose enters cells and is metabolised. The infused water enters both the ICF and ECF in proportion to their initial volumes.

The table below shows the results of infusing one litre of crystalloid solution in an average adult.

Crystalloid	↑ in ECF volume	↑ in ICF volume	Comment
Normal saline (0.9% NaCl)	+1,000	0	Na^+ remains in ECF
5% glucose	+333	+666	66% of TBW is ICF
0.45% saline	+666	+333	33% of TBW is ECF

Reprinted from Textbook of Anaesthesia, 3rd Edition. Aitkenhead AR, Smith G. (eds) 1996: 364, with permission from Elsevier.

6

How much fluid?

Your strategy should address the following issues:

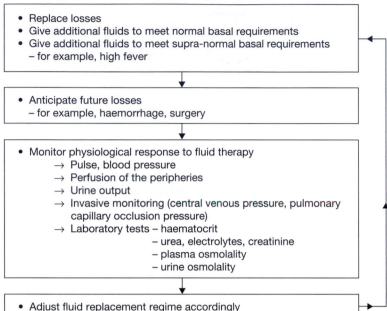

- Replace losses
- Give additional fluids to meet normal basal requirements
- Give additional fluids to meet supra-normal basal requirements
  – for example, high fever

- Anticipate future losses
  – for example, haemorrhage, surgery

- Monitor physiological response to fluid therapy
  → Pulse, blood pressure
  → Perfusion of the peripheries
  → Urine output
  → Invasive monitoring (central venous pressure, pulmonary capillary occlusion pressure)
  → Laboratory tests – haematocrit
                    – urea, electrolytes, creatinine
                    – plasma osmolality
                    – urine osmolality

- Adjust fluid replacement regime accordingly

Basal fluid requirements can be calculated from the **'4 – 2 – 1 rule'** (Table 6.3).

Table 6.3 **Basal requirements**

Body weight	Fluid/h
First 10 kg	4 ml/kg
Second 10 kg	2 ml/kg
Subsequent kg	1 ml/kg

For example a 25 kg person would need $(10 \times 4) + (10 \times 2) + (5 \times 1) = 65$ ml/h.

Full stomach

Vomiting is an active process that occurs in the lighter planes of anaesthesia, but regurgitation is a passive process that can happen at any time. If the stomach is full and the barrier pressure is exceeded (barrier pressure is the difference between the pressure exerted by the lower oesophageal sphincter and the intragastric pressure) then regurgitation will occur. Abnormal anatomy (e.g. pharyngeal pouches, strictures and hiatus hernias) also predispose to regurgitation (see Chapter 12: Causes and treatment of aspiration).

Factors that delay gastric emptying and result in a full stomach:

Physiological	anxiety
	pain
	trauma
	pregnancy
Pathological	gastric obstruction
	muscular/neurological
	metabolic/endocrine
Pharmacological	drugs (e.g. alcohol, morphine)

The interval between ingestion and trauma, rather than period of fasting is the best indicator of the degree of gastric emptying, as emptying virtually ceases at the time of trauma. For example, a child who has sustained a fractured arm shortly after a meal should be treated as if he has a full stomach even if surgery is planned to occur 6 h later, due to pain, anxiety and opioid analgesic drugs. However, it is still prudent if possible to fast from solids for 6 h, breast milk for 4 h and clear fluids for 2 h (N.B. These guidelines are very strictly applied for elective surgery).

If in doubt it is safest to assume that the stomach is full. If a general anaesthetic is required, a technique that takes account of this is necessary (e.g. a rapid sequence induction).

Full stomach management

6

Empty stomach before anaesthesia	nasogastric tube prokinetics (not in acute bowel obstruction)
Decrease acid	neutralise (antacids) inhibit secretion (proton pump inhibitors/H_2-antagonists)
Anaesthetic	rapid sequence induction

Fitness for anaesthesia

Preoperative physical status is assessed using the ASA classification system, originally devised by the American Society of Anesthesiologists. There are five categories (I–V), with the addition of the postscript E indicating emergency surgery.

ASA grade	Physical status
I	Normally healthy
II	Mild systemic disease
III	Moderate systemic disease with functional limitation
IV	Severe systemic disease that is a constant threat to life
V	Moribund patient not expected to survive 24 h, with or without an operation

The ASA grade is not a sensitive predictor of anaesthetic mortality and is applied inconsistently between anaesthetists, but correlates reasonably well with outcome. However, it does not include all aspects of anaesthetic and surgical risk. There is no allowance for extremes of age, although this, together with smoking and late pregnancy are often taken as criteria for a grade of at least ASA II. Nevertheless, it is useful and should be applied to all patients presenting for surgery and anaesthesia.

Pregnancy

Pregnant patients may occasionally present with acute surgical problems unrelated to pregnancy (e.g. trauma, appendicitis). Goals are to maintain the pregnant state and ensure the best outcome for mother and baby by maintaining placental perfusion and oxygenation. Attempts should be made to avoid maternal hypotension, hyperventilation, hypoxia, pain or anxiety. Liaise with the obstetric department. External fetal heart monitoring is feasible after 18 weeks and should be undertaken in the perioperative period. This can also reassure the mother, as non-obstetric surgery during pregnancy carries a significant risk of spontaneous abortion. From the 2nd trimester aorto-caval compression, when the gravid uterus compresses the great vessels against the lumbar vertebral bodies in the supine position, can cause hypotension by decreasing venous return to the heart. Patients should be transported and positioned on the operating table with a 15°–45° left lateral tilt or wedge. Advice should also be taken from the radiology department on the risk-benefit ratio of any investigation that involves X-rays. The majority of anaesthetic drugs are safe in pregnancy. Morphine can be used as an analgesic but may cause respiratory depression in the baby. Long-acting benzodiazepines should be avoided as they may sedate the fetus. Acid aspiration prophylaxis should be prescribed, as should graduated compression stockings (pregnancy is a hypercoaguable state). Early mobilisation should be encouraged.

6

Perioperative phase

Careful preparation of the patient and equipment should allow for all eventualities associated with the problems mentioned above, in addition to any discovered by the preoperative check.

Preparation
Analgesia
Rehydration with fluid resuscitation

Induction of anaesthesia
Rapid sequence induction:
Prior to the start of a rapid sequence induction the following requirements must be present:

1. A skilled assistant to apply cricoid pressure

2. A tilting trolley

3. Adequate suction

4. A means to ventilate the patient

5. A light source and equipment for intubation (including a variety of different sized endotracheal tubes)

6. The ability and means for a failed intubation drill!

The aim of the rapid sequence induction is to minimise the time between induction of anaesthesia, which abolishes protective airway reflexes and can lead to aspiration of acid passively regurgitated from the stomach, and the placement of a cuffed endotracheal tube that protects the airway. The patient is 'pre-oxygenated' with 100% oxygen for 3 min, which aims to fully saturate haemoglobin and increase oxygen reserve in the lungs. Hence, if there are any problems ventilating the patient after induction, there is time for the induction agent and muscle relaxant to wear off before profound hypoxaemia develops. Patients with high oxygen consumption (sepsis, neonates), lung disease or ventilation-perfusion mismatch (shunt caused by pulmonary embolus, atelectasis, obesity, neonates) will not have a great capacity to increase oxygen reserve despite preoxygenation.

The next stage is to induce anaesthesia using thiopentone or propofol, with suction to hand in the event of acid regurgitation. The anaesthetist's assistant then applies firm downward pressure to the cricoid cartilage of the larynx, which forms a complete ring around the trachea and lower larynx. Hence the posterior aspect of the cricoid cartilage compresses the oesophagus against the body of the sixth cervical vertebra, preventing passive regurgitation from the stomach. The rapid onset, rapid offset depolarising muscle relaxant suxamethonium is administered to facilitate placement of the endotracheal tube. Suitable intubating conditions develop within thirty seconds, however neuromuscular function returns in 3–5 min

6

so that protective airway reflexes will return and breathing recommence should it not be possible to intubate or ventilate the patient. Once the cuff of the endotracheal tube is inflated the airway is relatively safe from acid aspiration, although leakage can occur around the cuff (and children's larynxes are too narrow to accommodate a cuff) so if a full stomach is likely it should still be emptied by means of a wide bore orogastric tube.

Induction of anaesthesia for routine surgery, emergency surgery where there is little risk of aspiration, or if there are contraindications to using suxamethonium, does not follow the 'rapid sequence' protocol. The induction agent is likely to be propofol, with neuromuscular blockade achieved by a non-depolarising muscle relaxant (e.g. atracurium) if intubation or a long period of artificial ventilation is planned. The anaesthetist might otherwise use a laryngeal mask to secure the airway, which is less invasive and associated with fewer complications than intubation, but provides no protection against aspiration. In fact, when a laryngeal mask is *in situ*, it forms a seal over the oesophagus and larynx, so might make aspiration more likely if regurgitation occurs. Hence, anaesthetists only use the laryngeal mask in patients who represent very little or no risk of gastric regurgitation.

Failed intubation

Occasionally it is not possible to visualise the vocal cords on laryngoscopy and thus intubation can prove difficult or impossible. This is most likely to occur in patients with abnormal anatomy of the face, teeth, mouth or larynx, poor neck movements, limited mouth opening or pregnant women. This scenario becomes a life-threatening emergency if it is also not possible to ventilate, and consequently oxygenate the lungs – hence the use of short acting muscle relaxants in emergencies. Anaesthetists have many different means of assessing the likelihood of a patient having a difficult airway, but none are highly specific or sensitive. If a patient's airway appears to present a particular challenge, the anaesthetist may elect to undertake fibre-optic assisted nasotracheal intubation under local anaesthetic, with the patient awake and thus maintaining airway reflexes.

6

Incidence of failed intubation:	
General anaesthetic population	1 in 2,500
Obstetric population	1 in 250
'Can't ventilate, can't intubate'	Extremely rare but life threatening ? 1 in 10,000 to 1 in 1,000,000

Postoperative phase

Provision for postoperative monitoring, analgesia and fluid therapy is the responsibility of the anaesthetist. Consideration of the need for intensive or high dependency care postoperatively is best made at the earliest opportunity. If done preoperatively it allows easier organisation and explanation to patients and relatives.

NCEPOD

The National Confidential Enquiry into Peri-Operative Deaths (NCEPOD) is an ongoing study originally commissioned by the Association of Anaesthetists of Great Britain and Ireland and the Royal College of Surgeons of England. It was first published in 1987 as CEPOD. The first national Report (1989) focused on children under 10 years, and subsequent Reports focused on other particular aspects of surgery and anaesthesia.

General findings and recommendations have included the following:

■ most deaths occur in the elderly and sickest patients

■ overall care is good, but there are identifiable deficiencies

- inadequate consultation of senior surgeons and anaesthetists before emergency surgery

- inadequate communication between surgeons and anaesthetists

- inadequate supervision of locum and junior staff

- inappropriate surgery in 'hopeless cases'

- inadequate DVT prophylaxis

- surgeons should not operate outside their subspecialty

- inadequate preoperative resuscitation and optimisation

- inappropriate operating at night

- insufficient emergency operating, ICU and HDU resources

- poor quality and availability of medical notes/records

■ the need for post-mortem examinations, audit and morbidity/mortality reviews has been repeatedly stressed

The continued aim of NCEPOD is to reduce the mortality of surgery via retrospective analysis of perioperative deaths.

6

Key points

1. A successful outcome after emergency surgery requires thorough assessment and planning.

2. Accurate fluid therapy involves assessment of normal volumes and individual basal requirements, with accurate observation of losses.

3. Accurate, adequate and prompt fluid resuscitation is essential.

4. Predicting airway difficulty and having an alternative plan for the 'can't intubate can't ventilate' scenario is the only safe way to approach anaesthesia for the patient with a full stomach.

Further reading

Aitkenhead AR, Smith G. (eds) Textbook of Anaesthesia, 3rd edn. Churchill Livingstone, Edinburgh, 1996:361–371 & 519–532.

Boldt J. Volume replacement in the surgical patient – does the type of solution make a difference? Br J Anaesth 2000 Jun; 84(6):783–793.

Pre-operative Assessment – The Role of the Anaesthetist. Association of Anaesthetists, London, 2001. www.aagbi.org.

6

7

Perioperative fluid management

Iain MacKenzie

In health, fluid and electrolyte balance is tightly and effectively regulated by numerous homeostatic mechanisms. But in the elderly, sick, and those being prepared for, undergoing, or recovering from, surgery, these homeostatic mechanisms are either not functioning well, or, at all. For these patients, competent management of fluid and electrolyte balance plays a very significant contribution in determining a successful outcome.

The most pragmatic approach is to initially consider the issues of fluid *volume* and fluid *composition* separately, combining the respective requirements into an intravenous fluid prescription to cover each 24 h period.

Volume

Water is constantly lost from the body as urine, with smaller quantities lost from the lungs, mouth, skin and in faeces (so-called 'insensible' losses). The total is usually estimated as 1 ml/kg per hour with an additional 0.3 ml/kg per hour for every °C in body temperature above 37°C. Gastro-intestinal secretions (about 7,600 ml in all) are normally reabsorbed, but when lost in vomit, diarrhoea or naso-gastric aspirates, must be taken into account and replaced. Fluid may also be *effectively* lost from the intra-vascular space to other fluid spaces, for example the transcellular fluid. These losses are easily overlooked, and difficult to estimate, because the fluid does not leave the body but remains trapped in body cavities as ascites, pleural effusions, fluid-filled loops of bowel, or as oedema in the interstitial space ('third space' losses). Consequently effective fluid balance cannot be achieved by calculation alone, but needs to be adjusted by looking for clinical and laboratory evidence of over- and under-hydration (see Table 7.1). The baseline calculation would therefore be composed as follows:

Baseline calculation for **daily** fluid requirement
(a) Urinary and insensible losses **1 ml/kg/h** *multiplied by* **patient's weight (kg)** *multiplied by* **24 hours**
plus
(b) Extra losses for pyrexia (if patient's temperature >37°C) **(Temperature in °C −37)** *multiplied by* **0.3 ml/kg/h** *multiplied by* **24 hours**
plus
(c) Measured gastrointestinal losses
plus
(d) Adjustment for previous over- or underhydration
plus
(e) Estimated 'third space' losses

7

The sum of (a), (b), (c) and (d) above represent 'maintenance' volume, and providing the rate of loss is not too high, the burden is shared equally between all body compartments and can therefore be replaced in a 1:1 ratio by water, which will also distribute itself in the same way. Where fluid losses are not shared equally between the body compartments, such as when intra-vascular losses are brisk or caused by movement of volume from the intra-vascular to the 'third space' (e.g. (e) above), then consideration needs to be given to the way intravenous fluids are distributed in order to estimate the volumes required for 'resuscitation'.

Table 7.1 **Clinical and laboratory signs of fluid under- and over-replacement**

Dehydration	Fluid overload
Dry mucous membranes	Peripheral oedema
Sunken eyes	Pulmonary oedema (râles and/or end-inspiratory crepitations, hypoxaemia, tachypnoea, pleural effusion, 'bat's wing' shadowing on plain chest radiograph)
Skin 'tenting' in the elderly	Elevated jugular venous pressure
Oliguria (urine output less than 0.5 ml/kg per hour)	S3 gallop on cardiac auscultation
Contracted/absent veins on the dorsum of the hands	Orthopnoea
Absent jugular venous pulsation or low central venous pressure	Hyponatraemia
Postural hypotension	
Cold peripheries	
Hypotension and tachycardia	
Hypernatraemia	
Increased serum urea: creatinine ratio	
Urinary sodium <20 mmol/l	
Urine osmolality over 900 mOsmol/kg	

7

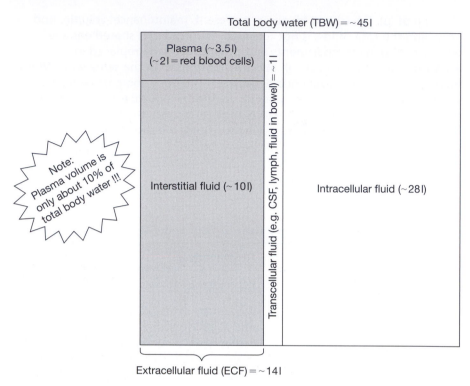

Fig. 7.1 Typical distribution of fluid in a 70 kg adult male.

Approximately 70% by weight of a lean adult man (less in females) is water, the exact proportion depending on the body proportion of fat, which has little water. In the average patient a more realistic proportion would be 55–60%. Approximately two thirds of body water is intracellular (46% by weight). The remaining third is divided between interstitial and transcellular fluids (lymph, cerebrospinal fluid, etc, 75% or 17% by weight), and intravascular fluid which accounts for 25%, or 6% by weight (see Figure 7.1).)

The intracellular fluid compartment is separated from the intravascular and interstitial fluid compartments by the cell membrane, which is freely permeable to water alone. The intravascular compartment is separated from the interstitial compartment by inter-cellular tight junctions of the capillary endothelium, whose permeability to water and small ions varies depending on the tissue in question and its pathological state. The distribution of intravenous fluids between the three compartments (intra-vascular, interstitial and intra-cellular) will depend on the effect the fluid has on the intra-vascular hydrostatic pressure and the plasma oncotic pressure. This can be seen in the annotated Figures 7.2 and 7.3.

7

Traditional view of fluid absorption in the capillary with filtration at the arteriolar end and absorption at the venular end. The net effect is a small degree of filtration with return via lymph.

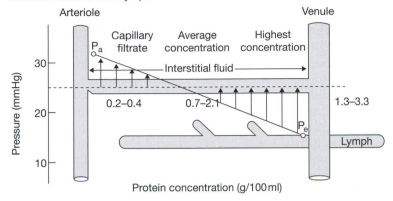

Fig. 7.2 Filtration-reabsorption pattern along the length of an 'average' capillary. Traditional view. Reproduced with permission from Folkow B, Neil E. Circulation, London: Oxford University Press, 1977.

Modern view emphasising the importance of interstitial forces. Predominantly filtration along entire length of the capillary. The net effect is greater filtration than with traditional view, again with return via lymph.

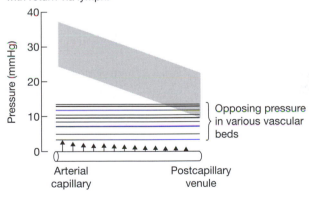

Fig. 7.3 Modern view. Reproduced with permission from Levick JR, 1995, Changing Perspectives on Microvascular Fluid Exchange. In: Jordan N, Marshall J, eds. Cardiovascular Regulation. © The Physiological Society.

Infusion of solutions that do not contain large molecules (referred to as 'crystalloids'), will cause an increase in capillary hydrostatic pressure and a fall in plasma oncotic pressure and will therefore distribute evenly within the extra-cellular space. Providing these solutions are isotonic to plasma water and interstitial fluid they will remain in the extra-cellular space, whilst hypotonic solutions will also distribute into the intra-cellular space and hypertonic solutions will draw water from within the intra-cellular compartment (see Table 7.2). Solutions that contain large molecules of gelatin (Haemaccel®, Gelofusine®), starch (eloHAES®, HAES-steril®) or dextran are known as 'colloids' and do not cause a reduction in plasma oncotic pressure when infused. These solutions therefore tend initially to remain within the intra-vascular space and in the short term (3–5 h) cause an increase in circulating volume in a 1:1 ratio. Eventually, however, the macromolecules of gelatin, starch or dextran are degraded, excreted by the kidney or taken up by the reticulo-endothelial system and the remaining fluid distributed across the whole extra-cellular space. In fact, to achieve a 500 ml increase in circulating volume requires only 500 ml of colloid, but requires 2,000 ml of isotonic crystalloid and 4,500 ml of 5% dextrose. Crystalloid solutions are therefore preferred for 'maintenance' fluids, colloids are suitable for rapid corrections in non-haemorrhagic

Table 7.2 Composition of common intravenous fluids

Fluid	Sodium	Potassium	Chloride	Bicarbonate	Calcium	Tonicity	pH	Osmolarity
0.9% sodium chloride ('normal saline')	150	–	150	–	–	↑		300
0.45% sodium chloride ('half-strength normal saline')	77	–	77	–	–	↓		
5% dextrose	–	–	–	–	–	↓↓↓	4	278
Dextrose-saline (4% dextrose, 0.18% sodium chloride)	30	–	30	–	–	↓↓		
Hartmann's solution	131	5	111	29	2	→	6	278
Haemaccel®	145	5.1	145	–	6.25	→		
Gelofusine®	154	0.4	125	–	–	↑	7.4	274
Hydroxyethyl starch (HAES-steril®, eloHAES®, Hespan®)	154	–	154	–	–	↑		308

↑ = Hypertonic; → = isotonic; ↓ = hypotonic.

7

intravascular volume deficits, whilst haemorrhagic losses are best replaced by a combination of packed red blood cells (PRBC) and colloids in a ratio of 4 volumes of PRBC to 3 volumes colloid.

Electrolytes

Sodium

In health, the body achieves electrolyte balance by matching the absorption and/or retention of electrolytes to urinary and faecal losses, with normal requirements calculated as 1 mmol/kg per day of sodium. Under normal circumstances the daily requirement for sodium and water is met by a solution containing about 42 mmol/l of sodium. As no such solution exists, this is best approximated by dextrose-saline (Table 7.2).

In the postoperative period, stress and pain both cause the non-osmotic release of anti-diuretic hormone, resulting in the re-absorption of water from the collecting duct and the excretion of lower volumes of more concentrated urine. Confusion can also arise because postoperative oliguria may be a sign of intra-vascular volume depletion arising from an early postoperative complication.

As serum sodium concentration reflects the ratio of extracellular sodium to extracellular water, abnormalities of sodium concentration cannot indicate whether the defect is one of sodium balance, water balance or both. Therefore fine-tuning of the patient's sodium requirements will depend on an independent assessment of the patient's fluid status (see Table 7.1), the serum sodium concentration and inspection of Table 7.2. In the perioperative period the commonest abnormalities of serum sodium concentration are due to inappropriate intravenous fluid therapy.

Symptomatic hypo- and hypernatraemia are medical emergencies that need careful management.

Symptoms of hypo- or hypernatraemia	
Hyponatraemia	**Hypernatraemia**
Headache	Thirst
Confusion	Confusion
Coma	Coma
Convulsions	Symptoms of intracerebral haemorrhage
Nausea	

7

Table 7.3 Diagnosis of sodium and water disorders

	Hypovolaemia	Euvolaemia	Oedema
Hyponatraemia	Sodium deficit +++ Water deficit ++	Sodium deficit + Water deficit 0	Sodium over-load + Water over-load ++
Hypernatraemia	Sodium deficit ++ Water deficit +++	Sodium over-load + Water deficit 0	Sodium over-load ++ Water over-load +

Over-correction or over-rapid correction can cause significant morbidity, most notably central pontine myelinolysis in the case of severe acute hyponatraemia. These patients are best managed in a high-dependency or intensive care setting.

Patients with severe symptomatic hyponatraemia should receive small volumes of either hypertonic or isotonic saline solution to increase serum sodium at ≤2 mmol/l per hour until the neurological symptoms have subsided, but without increasing the serum sodium concentration more than 12 mmol/l in the first 24 h. The serum sodium concentration should increase by slightly less in subsequent periods of 24 h. In the postoperative patient, the commonest cause of hyponatraemia is water retention rather than deficiency of sodium.

Patients with severe hypernatraemia should receive half-normal saline rather than solutions containing glucose. Glycaemic control is frequently abnormal and a glucose load increases renal free-water clearance by acting as an osmotic diuretic. As with hyponatraemia, hypernatraemia should be corrected gradually, aiming for a decrease of less than 0.5 mmol/l per hour during the first 24 h and even more slowly on subsequent days, with a serum sodium concentration not below 150 mmol/l in under 72 h.

Potassium

With normal renal function, total body potassium is regulated by renal loss or retention of potassium, as required by a dietary intake of 0.5–1 mmol/kg per day, although much less potassium is required in the 24 h following surgery due to the intense catabolism provoked by the surgical insult and uncertain renal function. Whilst maintenance of serum potassium concentrations in the range of 4.0–4.5 mmol/l are optimum, care should be taken in patients with impaired renal function or those requiring large quantities of packed red blood cells (which contain about 20 mmol of potassium per bag).

Hypokalaemia usually arises from fluid lost as diarrhoea (pathological or iatrogenic), vomiting or from enteric fistulae. As 98% of the body's potassium is intracellular patients can be suffering from severe potassium depletion even if their plasma potassium concentration is normal. Severe potassium depletion is usually accompanied by acid urine and very low urinary potassium concentrations. Correction of severe hypokalaemia requires the insertion of a central venous catheter and close monitoring by experienced staff in a high dependency or critical care area, as concentrated potassium solutions are irritant to peripheral veins and may precipitate ventricular arrhythmias.

Recommended reading

Mackenzie I. Assessment and management of fluid and electrolyte balance. Surgery 2002; 20: 121–126.

Park GR, Roe PG. Fluid Balance and Volume Resuscitation for Beginners. Greenwich Medical Media, London 2000.

7

8

Perioperative management of coagulation

Andy Johnston

8

This chapter will discuss the following aspects of coagulation

■ Coagulation pathway

■ Coagulation studies

■ Anticoagulants

■ Blood products

■ Common coagulation problems

The coagulation pathway

The interpretation of coagulation studies, patient anticoagulation and the correction of coagulation problems are made so much easier if one has a good understanding of the coagulation pathway.

Damage to a blood vessel wall initiates a series of steps to stop the bleeding, this involves three main mechanisms:

1. Vasoconstriction (sympathetic stimulation and vasoactive amines released from platelets)

2. Formation of a temporary platelet plug

3. Formation of a definitive fibrin clot by way of the clotting cascade

The coagulation pathway involves many circulating factors in a cascade mechanism; each factor, when activated, activates the next in turn (see fig. 8.1). All the clotting factors are produced in the liver except VIII and von Willebrand's Factor (vWF). The intrinsic pathway is initiated by the exposure of blood to collagen; the extrinsic pathway is initiated by thromboplastin released from damaged tissues. Both the intrinsic and extrinsic pathways activate the common pathway resulting in a tight fibrin clot.

Various mechanisms exist to prevent clotting and to limit clotting. The following are important to the understanding of coagulation problems and anticoagulation:

1. Fibrinolytic system

When clot forms, circulating plasminogen binds to fibrin and is converted to plasmin, which degrades fibrin into fibrin degradation products (FDPs). Activation involves XII, XI, kallikrein and kinins. FDPs inhibit clot formation by competing for fibrin polymerisation sites and interfering with platelet and thrombin function.

2. Antithrombin III

This is a circulating plasma protein which, after binding with heparin (either endogenous or exogenous) inactivates thrombin (factor II), and factors IXa, Xa, XIa and XIIa.

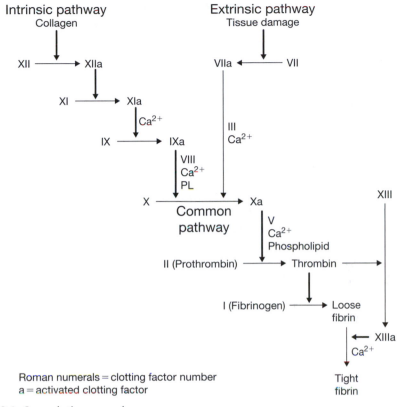

Fig. 8.1 Coagulation cascade.

Coagulation studies

The following coagulation tests are commonly performed by the haematology laboratory. A basic clotting screen will involve a full blood count (to give a platelet count), prothrombin time (PT) and activated partial thromboplastin time (APTT). Further tests can be requested as necessary.

■ Prothrombin Time (PT)
Citrated plasma and calcium are added to tissue thromboplastin to test the extrinsic pathway and the common pathway. The normal is 12–15 s. The international normalised ratio (INR) is the ratio of the sample time to a standard and it is used to monitor warfarin therapy. An INR <1.5 is usually required for surgery. PT increases in deficiency of factors V, VII and X, hypofibrinogenaemia, hypoprothrombinaemia, Vitamin K deficiency, disseminated intravascular coagulation (DIC), warfarin therapy, high levels of FDPs and hepatic failure.

■ Activated Partial Thromboplastin Time (APTT)
Plasma, phospholipid and calcium are added to kaolin. The APTT tests the intrinsic and common pathways. The normal is 35–40 s. The APTT ratio is

8

used to monitor heparin therapy. APTT increases in deficiency of factors XII, XI, IX, VIII, X, V and prothrombin, hypofibrinogenaemia, heparin therapy, high levels of FDPs, hepatic failure, DIC and vitamin K deficiency.

- Platelet Count
  Normal count is $150–400 \times 10^9/l$. A count of <50 results in easy bruising and is a contraindication to surgery. A count of <20 increases the risk of spontaneous bleeding. The platelet count does not always correspond to function; the bleeding time tests function. If the platelet count is normal and the bleeding time is increased then there may be a qualitative platelet defect, e.g. NSAID therapy or uraemia.

- Bleeding Time
  A standard incision is made on the forearm and a BP cuff is inflated around the upper arm to 40 mmHg. The wound is dabbed with filter paper every 30 s until the bleeding stops. Normal time is 2–9 min. It is prolonged in haemophilia A and B.

- Thrombin Time
  Exogenous thrombin is added to plasma, converting fibrinogen to fibrin. Normal time is 10–15 s. The thrombin time increases in DIC, heparin therapy, dysfibrinoginaemia or afibrinoginaemia and hepatic failure.

- Fibrinogen Assay
  Normal is 1.5–4 g/l. It is decreased in DIC.

- Fibrin Degradation Products (FDP)
  Levels reflect the level of fibrinolysis. FDPs are increased in DIC but may also be increased in other states such as trauma or inflammatory diseases. The normal is <10 mg/l.
- D Dimer
  This is only released during fibrinolysis and is more sensitive than FDPs. The normal is <500 ng/ml.

- Specific Factor Assays
  For example in haemophilia A, factor VIII activity should be greater than 50% for surgery.

Anticoagulants

The anticoagulants you are most likely to come across are warfarin, heparin and the low molecular weight heparins.

- Warfarin
  Warfarin competes with vitamin K in the hepatic synthesis of factors II, VII, IX and X. Warfarin is given orally and has a long half-life, lasting 4–5 days. The effects of warfarin are increased with a reduction in vitamin K (e.g. broad spectrum antibiotics), liver disease, liver microsomal enzyme inhibition and interference with protein binding, e.g. NSAIDs. Warfarin therapy is monitored by the PT and INR.

8

■ Heparin
Heparin accelerates the action of antithrombin III and inhibits platelet aggregation. Heparin has a fast onset and is short acting, with a half-life of approximately 90 min (increased in renal impairment) and is therefore best given by intravenous infusion. The effects of heparin last for 4–6 h after stopping an infusion. Heparin is monitored by the APTT ratio, although the thrombin time and PT also increase. Low molecular weight heparins inhibit factor Xa only and have a longer half-life of approximately 4 h. They have greater bioavailability than heparin and can be given as once daily injections on a per weight basis. In perioperative medicine you are most likely to come across low molecular weight heparins being used as prophylaxis against deep vein thrombosis (e.g. enoxaparin 2,000 units s.c. o.d.). Subcutaneous heparin can also be used for prophylaxis but there is some evidence that it is less efficacious and can increase the risk of bleeding.

Blood products

The blood products that are most likely to be used to correct coagulopathies are platelets, fresh frozen plasma (FFP) and cryoprecipitate.

■ Platelets
Each unit contains approximately 5×10^{10} platelets and increases the platelet count 1 h post transfusion by 5–10×10^9/l. Each unit comes from a single donor's unit of blood and it is normally pooled into bags of 5 units. Platelets are stored at 22–24°C with constant agitation. Transfusion is usually restricted to patients with a platelet count $<50 \times 10^9$/l unless platelet function is abnormal. Transfusion requires ABO compatibility. Platelets are normally given as 1 unit per 10 kg body weight (5–10 units for an average adult).

■ FFP
From each unit of donated blood 150–200 ml of plasma is obtained. After removing the platelets the plasma is frozen at −20°C. FFP needs to be thawed before use and must be used within 4 h of thawing. Transfused FFP is ABO compatible and Rh −ve if the recipient is a Rh −ve fertile female. FFP contains all the clotting factors at approximately 60% of normal levels. FFP is usually given at 10–15 ml/kg if the PT or APTT are greater than 1.5 times normal. FFP is used in liver disease, for the urgent reversal of warfarin, during massive blood transfusion and for DIC.

■ Cryoprecipitate
Cryoprecipitate is obtained by rapidly thawing FFP and it is then frozen and stored at −20°C. It is thawed immediately before use and must be used within 4 h. Cryoprecipitate is rich in factor VIII, fibrinogen and vWF. It is used in haemophilia A, von Willebrand's disease, DIC and liver

disease. Cryoprecipitate is normally given as 1.5–2 packs/10 kg body weight if the fibrinogen is less than 0.8 g/l. It is not normally group specific, but is Rh −ve if the recipient is a Rh −ve fertile female.

Common coagulation problems

The patient on warfarin

■ Elective surgery

Warfarin is a long acting anticoagulant (half-life is ∼30 h) and so all patients for elective surgery should have it stopped 3–5 days preoperatively and should have an INR checked immediately before surgery. The INR should be <1.5. The warfarin can normally be started again postoperatively. Before stopping the warfarin the condition requiring warfarinisation should be assessed and a decision made about alternative anticoagulation. For example, a patient warfarinised for atrial fibrillation would not normally require anticoagulation cover during the perioperative period, but a patient with a mechanical heart valve would. Heparin is most commonly used as the alternative anticoagulant. An infusion is normally started 24 h after the last dose of warfarin and it is stopped 6 h preoperatively. An APTT ratio should be checked immediately preoperatively and should be less than 1.5. The heparin is usually restarted 6 h postoperatively. The aim is to minimise the time period during which the patient is without anticoagulation (and therefore at risk), whilst allowing surgery to proceed without an increased risk of bleeding.

■ Emergency surgery

The anticoagulation needs reversing as soon as possible and this is normally done after discussion with the haematologists and anaesthetists. FFP and/or 1–10 mg of vitamin K are usually used. Vitamin K takes 12 h to work and may cause several weeks of upset to anticoagulation control. Anaphylactoid reactions may follow intravenous injection of vitamin K.

Liver disease

These patients may be coagulopathic because of decreased production of clotting factors and decreased absorption of lipid soluble vitamin K. There will be an increase in both PT and APTT. If surgery is required then FFP and vitamin K are used to correct the coagulopathy.

Disseminated intravascular coagulopathy (DIC)

DIC is the pathological activation of coagulation by a disease process leading to fibrin clot formation, consumption of platelets and coagulation factors and secondary fibrinolysis. There will be an elevated PT and APTT, thrombocytopaenia, reduced fibrinogen and raised FDPs and D dimer. Microangiopathic haemolysis leads to an increase in lactate dehydrogenase (LDH) and a reduced haptoglobin. The treatment of DIC is complicated but involves correcting the underlying problem, FFP, platelets and cryoprecipitate.

Massive transfusion

This will be discussed in 'Chapter 13: Transfusion and blood products'.

Others

For example von Willebrand's disease (autosomal dominant condition leading to abnormal synthesis of vWF and therefore decreased platelet adhesion and factor VIII deficiency), haemophilia A (Factor VIII deficiency), haemophilia B (Factor IX deficiency) and thrombocytopaenia (especially if immune in origin) will all need discussion with haematologists and anaesthetists before surgery.

9

Perioperative management of steroid therapy

Fraz Mir and Michael Lindop

Introduction

Glucocorticoids are powerful anti-inflammatory and immunosuppressive drugs that are used for a host of medical conditions (e.g. allergic reactions, asthma, connective tissue and rheumatic diseases, nephrotic syndrome, leukaemias and lymphomas, chemotherapy induced nausea and vomiting etc). Patients may also be on them as *replacement therapy* for primary deficiency states such as Addison's disease, hypopituitarism or following adrenalectomy. Preoperatively, people on long-term glucocorticoids require careful assessment to decide if additional or increased dosage might be in order. Although this will almost always be the case, the area of perioperative steroid therapy is controversial and there is no proper consensus or firm evidence so as to determine the best course of action.

The importance of adequate cortisol production

The function of the *hypothalamo-pituitary-adrenal axis* (HPA) is crucial in humans:

- the adrenal glands normally produce approximately 30 mg of cortisol (equivalent to 7.5 mg prednisolone) per day
- this increases in response to the degree of *stress* (e.g. after major surgery the serum cortisol level is 2–3 times higher than after minor surgery, which is only slightly higher than the norm)
- if the adrenal cortex does NOT keep up with the demands induced by physiological stress, for example post surgery or during an acute illness, circulatory collapse and shock can ensue with potentially fatal consequences (acute adrenocortical insufficiency or so-called 'Addisonian crisis')
- acute adrenocortical insufficiency is a medical emergency and MUST be recognised early and treated accordingly (Box 1)
- conversely, unnecessary or excessive steroid therapy also has its drawbacks. Long-term problems are significant (Table 9.1), but not directly life-threatening. Excessive therapy over only 1–2 days is unlikely to cause harm

Cortisol production and steroid therapy

Patients on long-term glucocorticoid therapy (including high-dose steroid inhalation e.g. beclomethasone 1.5 mg/day) have suppressed cortisol secretion from the adrenal glands via negative feedback to the hypothalamo-pituitary-adrenal axis. Thus, they are particularly vulnerable to stressful situations (such as surgery) and will require extra glucocorticoids during that period in order to avoid the complications highlighted above. This is also why long-term steroid therapy must NEVER be stopped abruptly but rather withdrawn *gradually*.

Box 1 **Addisonian crisis**

■ Very 'unwell' patient in shock: bradycardia or tachycardia, hypotension, confusion, weakness, coma, abdominal pain, hypoglycaemia (also note a low serum sodium and high serum potassium)

■ Management:

- if feasible, send blood for later measurement of serum cortisol and ACTH
- hydrocortisone 100 mg intravenously STAT
- aggressive intravenous fluid resuscitation with boluses of colloid (e.g. Gelofusine 500 ml STAT) or crystalloid (e.g. 1 litre 0.9% NaCl over 1 h)
- monitor serum electrolytes and glucose carefully and treat accordingly
- continue with intravenous steroid therapy until condition resolves (e.g. 100 mg in every 6–8 h, then convert to oral prednisolone)
- treat the cause of the crisis (e.g. antibiotics for infection; re-instituting daily steroids for those on long-term therapy who stop abruptly)
- if no rapid clinical response, establish central venous pressure monitoring at an early stage and consider transfer to high dependency or intensive care unit
- fludrocortisone (e.g. 50 mg) may also be required if primary adrenal failure suspected

Table 9.1 **The effect of too much vs. too little glucocorticoids**

Too much	Too little
Cushingoid appearance	Addisonian appearance
hypertension	hypotension
hyperglycaemia	hypoglycaemia
hypokalaemia	hyperkalaemia
weight gain/obesity	weight loss
poor wound healing	myalgia
increased risk of infection/sepsis	'flu-like' symptoms
osteoporosis	arthralgia
peptic ulcer disease	abdominal pain
hirsutism	vitiligo
Associated with delayed recovery and greater morbidity postoperatively	*Associated with shock, resistance to catecholamines and death postoperatively*

Most people on long-term steroids take prednisolone orally. When oral intake is not possible (or absorption from the gut is questionable), hydrocortisone intravenously (4 times the prednisolone dose) is the preferred substitute. It is useful to have an idea of the equivalent anti-inflammatory doses of the commonly used corticosteroids.

prednisolone 5 mg	≡ hydrocortisone 20 mg
	≡ cortisone acetate 25 mg
	≡ methylprednisolone 4 mg
	≡ dexamethasone 750 mcg
	≡ betamethasone 750 mcg
	≡ triamcinolone 4 mg

Preoperative assessment

As for all patients planned to undergo surgery, a careful history is crucial in patients on long-term glucocorticoid therapy:

- the history should include a detailed drug history – the reason for steroid therapy, its duration and the dosage (call the GP if you need to!)
- the steroid treatment card that these patients often carry can be invaluable in such circumstances
- check the medical records to see what was done during a previous operation
- on examination, note evidence of a Cushingoid appearance, or hyperpigmentation associated with an Addisonian state – does the patient have a *Medic-Alert* bracelet or necklace?
- check for postural hypotension – remember that patients on steroid replacement therapy will often be on fludrocortisone as well to provide adequate mineralocorticoid activity
- ensure that urea and electrolyte levels (especially sodium and potassium), glucose and full blood count are measured
- further tests (such as a short Synacthen® test) can be used to gauge the level of adrenal suppression but the results are often delayed. Results are often difficult to interpret in stressed patients and add little to the decision to give additional steroids

How much additional steroids are required?

As a general rule, the consensus is that patients who have taken more than 10 mg prednisolone daily (or equivalent) for more than a week, in the 3 months prior to surgery, require extra glucocorticoids to cover the operation. However, many choose to give supplemental treatment to patients on steroids routinely rather than risk a precipitous fall in blood pressure during anaesthesia and subsequent acute adrenal insufficiency. The extra steroids are continued for a variable period, depending upon the individual circumstances. Often the start of an oral diet marks the end of the need for supplementation.

Table 9.2 **Suitable perioperative intravenous hydrocortisone dosage for patients on long-term corticosteroids**

Medical or surgical stress	Stress dose	Duration*
MINOR (e.g. inguinal hernia repair, colonoscopy, mild febrile illness, mild to moderate nausea, vomiting, gastroenteritis)	25 mg/day	1 day
MODERATE (e.g. total joint replacement, open cholecystectomy, hemicolectomy, significant febrile illness, pneumonia, severe gastroenteritis)	50–75 mg/day in divided doses	1–2 days
SEVERE (e.g. major cardiothoracic surgery, Whipple's procedure, liver resection, pancreatitis)	100–150 mg/day in divided doses	2–3 days
CRITICALLY ILL (e.g. sepsis induced hypotension, shock)	50–100 mg every 6–8 h or 0.18 mg/kg/h as an infusion PLUS 50 mg/day fludrocortisone	until shock resolved (may take several days), then cautiously withdraw

* In the absence of complications.
NB. REMEMBER to continue usual corticosteroid dose afterwards.
Adapted from a table in Further reading no. 3.

Additional perioperative steroid therapy depends on three major factors:

■ daily dosage of glucocorticoids – the higher the dose, the greater the severity of adrenal suppression

■ duration of glucocorticoid therapy – adrenal atrophy can occur as quickly as a week after starting treatment and can persist for years after it has been stopped

■ the degree of physiological stress the patient is to undergo (e.g. hernia repair vs. major cardiothoracic surgery)

Table 9.2 shows a suitable regimen for additional corticosteroid therapy. The doses are controversial and aim to reduce significant untoward effects of high dose steroids perioperatively (see Table 9.1). Higher doses have been used in the past.

If in doubt, it is always best to ask an endocrinologist!

Key points

1. The majority of patients on chronic steroid treatment will require steroid supplementation during acute illnesses and surgery.

2. Acute adrenocortical insufficiency is an often forgotten cause of circulatory collapse and shock.

3. Long-term steroid therapy should always be withdrawn gradually via a reducing dose regimen.

Further reading

1 Lindop MJ. Perioperative management of anticoagulants, corticosteroids and immunosuppression. Surgery 2002; 20:96a–96e.

2 Shaw M. When is perioperative 'steroid coverage' necessary? Cleve Clin J Med 2002 Jan; 69(1):9–11.

3 Kelley III JT and Conn DL. Perioperative management of the rheumatic disease patient. Bulletin on the Rheumatic Diseases 2002; 51(6).

4 Holte K, Sharrock NE and Kehlet H. Perioperative single-dose glucocorticoid administration: Pathophysiologic effects and clinical implications. J Am Coll Surg 2002; 195(5):694–712.

10

Perioperative management of endocrine disease

Dan Wheeler and Ingrid Wilkins

Patients with endocrine diseases presenting for surgery commonly have impaired physiological responses to anaesthesia and surgery. Endocrine disease may not be the primary indication for surgery, indeed it might not have been previously diagnosed so it is important to have a basic understanding of the conditions associated with, and complications that can arise from them. Endocrinopathies may in turn lead to or result from other comorbidities, for example hypothyroid patients have an increased incidence of ischaemic heart disease and some lung tumours secrete adrenocorticotrophic hormone (ACTH). Surgical trainees are primarily responsible for detecting, managing and optimising these diseases in conjunction with anaesthetists and endocrinologists. This chapter reviews the perioperative management of patients with endocrinopathies. (see Chapter 11: Perioperative management of diabetes)

10

Disorders of the thyroid gland

Thyroid disorders are common and are well controlled in the majority of patients. However, surgery and anaesthesia carry significant risks to patients with uncontrolled hypo- or hyperthyroidism (who may present for emergency surgery).

The thyroid gland secretes thyroxine (T4) and triiodothyronine (T3), which increase tissue metabolism and optimise cellular oxygen consumption. Thyroid activity is therefore the major determinant of metabolic rate. Release of T3 and T4 is controlled by thyroid-stimulating hormone (TSH), which is secreted by the anterior pituitary, which in turn is controlled by thyrotropin-releasing hormone (TRH) from the hypothalamus. This system is under negative-feedback control. Iodide is necessary to produce T3 and T4.

Goitres

Enlargement of the thyroid gland may be due to carcinoma, adenoma, iodine deficiency, autoimmune thyroiditis and thyrotoxicosis (secondary to pituitary hypersecretion of TSH). The presence of a goitre gives no clue as to the thyroid status of that patient, which must be ascertained by biochemical tests. However it is an important clinical finding and the patient should be carefully examined for signs of tracheal compression leading to respiratory embarrassment (which may only be present on exercising). Retrosternal goitres can cause tracheal compression or deviation, recurrent laryngeal nerve palsy or superior vena cava obstruction. Chest and thoracic inlet X-rays and indirect laryngoscopy are useful investigations in these patients providing the anaesthetist with information about potential airway and intubation difficulties. At induction, specialist fibre-optic intubation may be required.

Acute stridor and life-threatening airway obstruction may also develop after extubation. Causes include bilateral recurrent laryngeal nerve damage, haematoma or tracheomalacia (inspiratory collapse of a tracheal wall weakened by erosion of the tracheal cartilage). These problems usually present early, often in the recovery area. If the airway seems clear, pneumothorax should be considered.

Hypothyroidism (myxoedema)

Hypothyroidism is more common in women and in the elderly and circulating levels of T3 and T4 are low. Primary hypothyroidism is caused by intrinsic thyroid atrophy, autoimmune disease (e.g. Hashimoto's thyroiditis), drugs (e.g. amiodarone, lithium), or result from treatment of hyperthyroidism with radioactive iodine or surgery. TSH is raised. Secondary hypothyroidism, when TSH is low due to anterior pituitary failure, is rare.

Hypothyroid patients complain of feeling cold and lethargic, having poor appetite with weight gain, hoarse voice, depression and constipation. Examination may reveal hair loss (including the outer third of the eyebrow), bradycardia, low temperature, obesity, coarse and pallid skin and delayed tendon reflexes. The presence of these features does not correlate with the severity of hypothyroidism. Further investigation may reveal macrocytic anaemia, cardiomegaly, pericardial effusion and the ECG changes of ischaemic heart disease (caused by hyperlipidaemia).

Elective surgery should be postponed until the patient is euthyroid. A normal TSH level is the best indication of adequate treatment. However, the half-lives of T4 and T3 are relatively long ($t_{1/2}$ = 7 days and 1½ days respectively) and there may not be time to correct hypothyroidism before emergency surgery. Hypothyroid patients undergoing emergency surgery are at very high risk of coma, myocardial ischaemia, hypotension, hypoventilation, hypothermia, acidosis, hypoglycaemia and hyponatraemia leading to convulsions. Metabolism and excretion of drugs is impaired and regional anaesthetic techniques should be used whenever possible. If a general anaesthetic is required the drug doses are titrated very carefully and the patient is kept warm. Intravenous T3 should be given cautiously after seeking the opinion of an endocrinologist and with full monitoring. Sudden correction of hypothyroidism may precipitate myocardial ischaemia. Impaired cardiac contractility responds poorly to fluid replacement and inotropes in this condition. 'Hypothyroid coma' is precipitated by hypothermia, infection, stroke, surgery and general anaesthesia and requires admission to the intensive care unit. It has a 50% mortality.

Hyperthyroidism (thyrotoxicosis)

Thyrotoxicosis is most commonly caused by Graves' disease, an autoimmune disease mediated by thyroid-stimulating IgG immunoglobulins directed against the TSH receptor, resulting in hyperthyroidism. The autoimmune process involved in Graves' disease is typically directed to the soft tissues within the orbit resulting in periorbital

10

oedema, proptosis and ophthalmoplegia. Pretibial myxoedema is diagnostic but only seen in 5% of patients with the disease.

Other causes of hyperthyroidism include toxic uni- or multinodular goitres that produce T4 and T3 outside the influence of normal negative feedback mechanisms. Investigation will show raised T4 and/or T3 levels with low or undetectable TSH. Many of the clinical features of thyrotoxicosis are characterised by signs of sympathetic overactivity such as tremor, tachycardia, sweating, diarrhoea, palpitations, angina and breathlessness producing weight loss, fatigue and heat intolerance. The level of catecholamines is normal but the excess thyroid hormones seem to potentiate the action of the catecholamines. Examination may reveal tachycardia, atrial arrhythmias and signs of heart failure. An ECG will confirm and document arrhythmias.

Elective surgery should be postponed until the patient is euthyroid. Carbimazole and propylthiouracil can be used to reduce thyroid hormone production, but cause an increase in thyroid gland vascularity so are stopped 7–10 days before surgery. Then thyroid hormone production can be controlled by a large dose of iodine, which inhibits the iodination of thyroid hormones and reduces vascularity of the thyroid gland. β-blockers reduce peripheral conversion of T4 to T3 and improve the symptoms of thyrotoxicosis. Radioactive iodine can also be given to abolish thyroid activity, after which patients take thyroxine. Thyrotoxicosis can be associated with other autoimmune disease such as myasthenia gravis, which will also require investigation and treatment.

Unfortunately there may not be time to correct hyperthyroidism before emergency surgery. The patient's cardiovascular system is usually unstable and will require invasive monitoring. Esmolol, a short acting β-blocker, is a useful drug in this situation allowing the anaesthetist to control hypertension precisely and rapidly. A 'thyroid crisis' is a rare manifestation of severe hyperthyroidism and is triggered by infection or surgery. It presents with hyperthermia, life-threatening arrhythmias, cardiorespiratory failure, metabolic acidosis and coma. Treatment with iodine suppression and steroids is started immediately and admission to intensive care for cooling, sedation, ventilation and supportive measures should be arranged. Thyroid surgery has been performed under local anaesthetic infiltration in very high risk cases.

Disorders of the parathyroid glands

The four parathyroid glands lie adjacent to the superior and inferior poles of the thyroid although their exact location is very variable. In fact 6% of the population have less than four parathyroid glands. They are involved in calcium homeostasis and produce parathyroid hormone (PTH). PTH increases the concentration of calcium in the blood by increasing renal Ca^{++} reabsorption and releasing calcium from bone.

Primary, secondary and pseudo-hyperparathyroidism

A parathyroid adenoma secreting PTH is the commonest cause of primary hyperparathyroidism. Hypercalcaemia and hypophosphataemia are the biochemical findings and blood levels of intact (unmetabolised, active) PTH are high. Urinalysis reveals hypercalciuria (although PTH causes renal Ca^{++} reabsorption, high urinary calcium results from high blood levels) and phosphaturia. Hypercalcaemia is often an incidental finding, but patients may present with renal stones, peptic ulcers, pancreatitis, abdominal pain or psychiatric disturbance. Hypertension is a common finding. Rarely a hypercalcaemic crisis occurs with profound hypovolaemia, prerenal failure, cardiac arrhythmias and coma.

Hypercalcaemia is associated with dehydration and renal impairment and this must be corrected preoperatively with intravenous fluids. Calcium can then be lowered using frusemide (which decreases calcium reabsorption in the Loop of Henle). Central venous pressure (CVP) monitoring and a urinary catheter are useful to aid treatment as maintenance fluid requirements increase with the diuresis. If diuretics are given before adequate rehydration is achieved then the renal function will deteriorate. In severe cases of hypercalcaemia, bisphosphonates, corticosteroids, calcitonin, calcium resonium or even dialysis may be necessary. Hypertension, if present, should be controlled.

Intra-operative considerations include very careful patient positioning as decalcified bones fracture easily. Surgery may be prolonged, as the parathyroid glands are difficult to locate and often require histological confirmation that the correct tissue has been excised.

Secondary hyperparathyroidism describes parathyroid hyperplasia secondary to chronically low serum calcium levels, e.g. chronic renal failure. Biochemistry shows high serum phosphate with low or normal calcium levels and a raised intact PTH. Some patients in chronic renal failure require parathyroidectomy for symptom control, despite calcium supplements and low phosphate diets. Perioperative CVP monitoring is required because of impaired or absent renal function. Central lines can be inserted under direct vision by the surgeon after parathyroidectomy to avoid haematoma formation near the operative field.

Pseudo-hyperparathyroidism describes ectopic secretion of PTH, for example from a bronchial carcinoma and may be asymptomatic.

Hypoparathyroidism

The aetiology of hypoparathyroidism may be autoimmune or familial but is most commonly iatrogenic. The parathyroid glands are often inadvertently removed during thyroid or neck surgery. This group of patients are at risk of developing hypocalcaemia and hyperphosphataemia postoperatively. This may occur within hours or even months later. Hypocalcaemic patients may be agitated or describe parasthesiae, muscle cramps and spasms (Chvostek's sign – percussion over facial nerve causes facial spasm and Trousseau's sign – tourniquet inflated above arterial pressure causes carpopedal spasm). They are at risk of stridor, convulsions

10

and compromised cardiac output. These symptoms are exacerbated by low serum magnesium, which frequently coexists with hypocalcaemia. Intravenous calcium salts should be given carefully, especially to those with ischaemic heart disease. Magnesium supplements should also be given.

Disorders of the pituitary gland

Although pituitary surgery is likely to take place in specialist centres, pituitary disease causes many symptoms, so patients may present to any surgical speciality. For example, an acromegalic patient might need carpal tunnel decompression.

The anterior pituitary produces growth hormone (GH), TSH, adrenocorticotrophic hormone (ACTH), prolactin, sex hormones and melanocyte-stimulating hormone (MSH). The posterior pituitary secretes anti-diuretic hormone (ADH, vasopressin) and oxytocin. Pituitary tumours may over-secrete any of these hormones, possibly at the expense of the others, or if 'non-functioning' can cause global hypopituitarism. An endocrinologist will have assessed the pituitary function preoperatively. This chapter will concentrate on the perioperative problems encountered in three of the more common or serious pituitary diseases.

Acromegaly

Overproduction of GH in the adult causes soft tissue and some bony enlargement to give the classic appearance of heavy facial features with big hands and feet. Of more importance perioperatively are the enlargement of the tongue and thyroid, the hypertension and left ventricular hypertrophy with impaired ventricular function and the impaired glucose tolerance that accompany this condition. A careful assessment of cardiac function should be performed and blood pressure and blood glucose optimised preoperatively.

All aspects of airway management are more difficult in acromegaly. Facemask ventilation is made difficult by changes in facial anatomy and the large tongue. Pharyngeal and laryngeal tissue enlargement decreases the size of the laryngeal aperture and laryngoscopy and intubation can be difficult or impossible. Indirect laryngoscopy may be required as part of the preoperative airway assessment. These patients often have some degree of obstructive sleep apnoea, which may cause problems postoperatively (particularly if they have received opioids).

Diabetes insipidus (DI)

DI is characterised by passage of large volumes of dilute urine. In cranial DI, the production of ADH by the pituitary is reduced following head injury, neurosurgery or an intracranial tumour. Treatment is with the ADH analogue desmopressin. In nephrogenic DI, the distal renal tubules become unresponsive to circulating ADH, due to drugs like lithium and gentamicin and treatment is with thiazide diuretics. Large volumes (>2 ml/kg/h) of hypotonic urine (<300 mOsm/kg) are produced despite increased plasma osmolality (>295 mOsm/kg). Careful perioperative fluid management is required to avoid hypovolaemia and hypernatraemia.

Hypopituitarism

The pituitary gland is almost entirely surrounded by bone and so any tumour or growth within it will compress neighbouring cells reducing their normal secretory capacity. Hypopituitarism may also follow irradiation or surgery to the pituitary fossa, granulomatous disease or Sheehan's syndrome (ischaemic necrosis following obstetric haemorrhage). Secretion of any or all the hormones may be affected. In the perioperative setting the most important are secondary hypothyroidism (lack of TSH) and secondary hypoadrenalism (lack of ACTH). Abnormalities of these endocrine axes should be corrected before surgery.

These patients may be taking supplemental growth and sex hormones. Anyone who has ever received human derived growth hormone or who has had a human dural graft following surgery might have been exposed to prion disease and nursing and medical staff should take appropriate precautions.

10

Disorders of the adrenal glands

The adrenal glands lie on the superior pole of each kidney and comprise a medulla that secretes adrenaline and noradrenaline and a cortex, which has three zones. One secretes the mineralocorticoid hormone aldosterone, another secretes the glucocorticoid hormone cortisol and sex hormones are secreted from the inner zona.

Adrenocortical insufficiency

Primary disease of the adrenal cortex causes a lack of cortisol and aldosterone and may result from autoimmune disease, tuberculosis, metastatic infiltration, haemorrhage or infarction. Secondary insufficiency results from a failure of the anterior pituitary gland to secrete adequate ACTH, or sudden withdrawal of corticosteroid therapy. The normal adrenal response to physiological stress (e.g. illness or surgery) is to increase steroid production. Hypoperfusion or infarction of the adrenals during critical illness or major surgery may blunt this response and adrenocortical insufficiency may develop. The acute features are hypotension and electrolyte imbalance (hyponatraemia, hyperkalaemia, hypochloraemia, hypercalcaemia and hypoglycaemia). However it should be suspected when hypotension does not respond to fluid replacement or pressor agents. Many intensive care units routinely screen for this with an ACTH (Synacthen™) stimulation test. Treatment attempts to mimic the normal adrenal response to stress by administering corticosteroid during the period of physiological stress (2–3 days for straightforward surgery, longer

10

for an ICU admission). Mineralocorticoids sometimes need to be replaced separately. (see Chapter 11: Perioperative management of steroid therapy)

Cushing's syndrome

This syndrome describes the symptoms and signs of excess circulating glucocorticoids, usually resulting from corticosteroid replacement therapy. Other causes are adrenal adenoma/carcinoma or excessive ACTH production either by the pituitary (Cushing's disease) or an ectopic tumour (e.g. lung). Diagnosis is made by demonstrating raised 24-hour urinary free cortisol levels, or by means of a low dose dexamethasone suppression test.

Preoperatively, hypertension, hypokalaemia, hypernatraemia and diabetes mellitus may be evident and should be corrected or optimised. The drug metyrapone (an 11β-hydroxylase inhibitor) suppresses steroid synthesis and can be useful but the dose should be carefully titrated by an endocrinologist. Surgery can be technically difficult due to central obesity, which, combined with a proximal myopathy can cause respiratory problems postoperatively. Hypoxia and atelectasis can quickly lead to pneumonia in this group of immunocompromised individuals. Patients are also at increased risk of cardiac failure. Wound healing is impaired by high levels of steroid, hyperglycaemia and thin, fragile skin that bruises easily. Careful attention should be given to control of blood glucose and electrolyte balance throughout.

Secretagogue tumours or APUDomas

A group of rare tumours classified as APUDomas (they originate from amine precursor uptake and decarboxylation cells) also secrete hormones or polypeptides and amines that mimic hormone action. A very brief description of them is given here.

Phaeochromocytomas secrete noradrenaline (norepinephrine) and/or adrenaline (epinephrine) and/or dopamine and arise from the adrenal medulla (94%) or sympathetic nervous system (6%). They cause hypertension, ischaemia and tachyarrhythmias. Preoperative preparation includes α-adrenoceptor blockade followed by β-adrenoceptor blockade. These patients require an experienced anaesthetist and invasive monitoring before, during and after their anaesthetic as very dramatic swings in blood pressure can occur.

Carcinoid tumours arise from the terminal ileum in 85% of cases and secrete a range of vasoactive amines including 5-hydroxytryptamine (5-HT), kallikrein, prostaglandins and histamine. They can cause bronchospasm, flushing, sweating, hypertension, hypotension and diarrhoea. Preoperative treatment with octreotide or methyldopa can reduce amine secretion. Perioperatively, invasive monitoring is essential and use of histamine releasing drugs is avoided. Blood pressure remains labile for several days postoperatively and ICU care is appropriate.

Table 10.1 Other secretagogue tumours or APUDomas

	Organ affected	Hormone(s) secreted	Clinical features	Preoperative management	Perioperative management	Postoperative management
Insulinoma	β-cells of pancreas	Insulin	Fasting hypoglycaemia (commonly at night)	Careful attention to blood glucose and electrolyte levels, infusion of glucose and K^+	Diazoxide and verapamil are unpredictable and have unwanted adverse effects	
Glucagonoma	α-cells of pancreas	Glucagon	Diabetes mellitus, erythematous rash, diarrhoea, profound weight loss, glossitis, stomatitis, anaemia	Nutritional support and supplementation Antithrombotic agents due to ↑ risk of DVT Somatostatin analogues if hepatic metastases		
Gastrinoma (Zollinger-Ellison syndrome)	Duodenum, pancreas, ovary	Gastrin	Diarrhoea, steatorrhoea, acid reflux oesophagitis, pernicious anaemia	Proton pump inhibitors Correct clotting abnormalities (vitamin K absorption)	Nasogastric tube H₂-antagonists	
VIPoma	Body and tail of pancreas, autonomic nervous system	Vasoactive intestinal polypeptide	Profuse watery diarrhoea, hypotension, ileus, abdominal distension, tetany, ↓K^+, ↓Mg^{++}, ↓H^+	Replace profuse K^+-rich fluid losses Somatostatin analogues, steroids Control hypotension, may need pressors as VIP vasodilates H₂-antagonists control rebound gastric acid hypersecretion		
Somatostatinoma	δ-cells of pancreas	Somatostatin	Obstructive jaundice, gallstones, diabetes mellitus, steatorrhoea	Relieve obstructive jaundice with stent		

10

Table 10.2 **The categorisation of the multiple endocrine neoplasias**

	Other name	Tumour sites	Other features
MEN-1	Wermer syndrome	Anterior pituitary adenoma	Peptic ulcers
		Parathyroid adenoma	Adrenal and thyroid hyperfunction
		Pancreatic adenomas (especially gastrinomas)	May have associated carcinoid syndrome
MEN-2A	Sipple syndrome	Medullary carcinoma of thyroid	Parathyroid hyperplasia
		Phaeochromocytoma	↑incidence of meningiomas, gliomas
MEN-2B	Gorlin or Steinert syndrome	Very aggressive medullary carcinoma of thyroid	
MEN-3	Mucosal neuroma syndrome	Medullary carcinoma of thyroid	Neurofibromatosis or isolated neuromas of lips, tongue, buccal mucosa
		Phaeochromocytoma	Tall, thin stature often mistaken for Marfan's syndrome

Other APUDomas are less common and may arise from anterior pituitary, thyroid, adrenal, gastrointestinal, pancreatic, lung and carotid body tissue. They are summarised in Table 10.1.

Multiple endocrine neoplasia/adenomatosis (MEN)

In these autosomal dominant inherited syndromes patients have two or more endocrinopathies. They may present simultaneously or onset may be separated by as much as 10 years. For this reason diagnosis has been difficult, but discovery of the MEA-1 gene on chromosome 11 in 1997 has improved this. When treating a patient with an endocrinopathy is always worth considering that it may fit in to one of these syndromes (summarised in Table 10.2).

10

Further reading

Nicholson G, Burrin J and Hall GM. Perioperative steroid supplementation. Anaesthesia 1998; 11:1091–1104.

Postgraduate educational issue: Endocrine and metabolic disorders in anaesthesia and intensive care. Br J Anaesth 2000; 85:1–183.

10

11

Perioperative management of diabetes

Mike Masding and Wendy Gatling

Introduction

Diabetes mellitus is a very common disease, affecting 3–4% of the population, with an increasing prevalence with age. People with diabetes will be commonly encountered on surgical wards with standard surgical problems. On the vascular unit, the increased risk of peripheral vascular disease associated with diabetes means that diabetic patients are frequently admitted for surgical procedures on the lower limb.

Admission to hospital is stressful and this change in daily routine, exercise and food patterns is likely to have a major impact on the control of plasma glucose levels in people with diabetes. The maintenance of good glycaemic control in people with diabetes is important in the perioperative period. Poor glycaemic control impairs the response to infection and slows wound healing. Raised plasma glucose levels may be the first indicators of a problem such as occult infection.

This chapter discusses measures to ensure good glycaemic control whilst undergoing surgical procedures and in the postoperative period.

Preoperative preparation

11

Preoperative assessment

■ Good preoperative diabetes control helps to reduce postoperative complications.

■ Patients attending the preoperative assessment clinic may have undiagnosed diabetes. Check random plasma glucose on all patients at preadmission assessment and be particularly suspicious if they have recurrent fungal infections, a history of thirst, polyuria, nocturia or weight loss. Check also for peripheral vascular disease. If random plasma glucose ≥8 mmol/l, organise further investigations. In the presence of symptoms, fasting plasma glucose ≥7 mmol/l, or random plasma glucose ≥11.1 mmol/l are diagnostic of diabetes (NB: A fasting glucose <7 mmol/l does not exclude diabetes. If clinical suspicion is high but initial test is not diagnostic, organise an oral glucose tolerance test).

■ In patients with preexisting diabetes, check HbA1c in the preadmission clinic and discuss with the Diabetes Nurse Specialist or Diabetes team if diabetes control needs improvement prior to surgery. This blood test is an indicator of glycaemic control over the previous 8 weeks and is used to assess the success of treatment. The normal range may vary between laboratories but a reasonable assessment prior to surgery is HbA1c <6.5% excellent control, HbA1c 6.5–8.0% adequate control and HbA1c >8.0% poor control.

■ Patients with diabetes have a high incidence of hypertension, so blood pressure should be checked and appropriate treatment started. Again, discuss with the Diabetes team or GP if blood pressure control needs improvement prior to surgery.

■ People with diabetes have a high incidence of ischaemic heart disease and left ventricular failure. Silent myocardial ischaemia is not uncommon and the anaesthetist should be informed and further investigation instigated as required.

Preoperative planning

■ Ensure the patient is first on the list, so that minimal disruption is caused to their routine – the exceptions are:

- Emergency case.

- Dirty wounds.

- More than one diabetic on the list.

■ Identify diabetic patients and make the anaesthetists aware.

■ Discuss with the patient how their diabetes will be managed. Patients often have considerable knowledge and expertise in managing their diabetes and dislike the lack of control over their diabetes treatment when they are in hospital. If the patient is knowledgeable, allow them to monitor and adjust the dose of insulin. If there are any problems, or if the patient requests it, involve the Diabetes team at an early stage.

11

How to manage diabetes during surgery

The most important factor dictating perioperative diabetes management is how long the patient will be fasting before surgery and how quickly they will be able to eat after surgery. For the purposes of this chapter, the term minor surgery describes an operation where the patient will be allowed to eat within a few hours and major surgery refers to an operation where the patient will remain 'nil by mouth' for more than 6 h following surgery.

Patients have been divided into three groups depending on their mode of treatment, offering a simple and safe way to manage patients. These guidelines have been developed over years of treating patients with diabetes during surgery – the Diabetes team is always available for further advice.

(i) Basic principles during the operation

■ Monitor capillary glucose 2–4 hourly.

■ Avoid hypoglycaemia, as patients are unable to recognise and treat it.

■ Aim for mean blood glucose of 5–7 mmol/l.

(ii) Diet only therapy

■ The patient fasts as per normal anaesthetic instructions and capillary glucose is monitored four times a day (before meals and before bed).

■ People with diabetes treated by diet alone do not become hypoglycaemic, so monitor glucose to ensure that good glycaemic control is maintained.

- Intravenous dextrose must be avoided as fluid replacement as plasma glucose will rise.
- If capillary glucose remains >10 mmol/l for >24 h, the diabetic team should be involved to instigate more intensive treatment.

(iii) Patients on tablet only therapy

- Patients taking long acting hypoglycaemic drugs like glibenclamide may develop prolonged hypoglycaemia if fasted. If possible, change tablets to short acting (e.g. gliclazide, glipizide) preoperatively.

Minor surgery – (No restrictions to eating in the postoperative period)

- Omit tablets on the morning of surgery and give postoperatively with a light meal.
- Postoperatively, record capillary glucose 4 hourly until full recovery from anaesthesia.

Major surgery – (Restrictions to eating in the postoperative period)

Morning list	Afternoon list
Fast from midnight	Fast from 0800 h
Omit tablets	Usual tablets at breakfast**
Start glucose insulin infusion at 0700 h*	Allow usual breakfast Start glucose insulin infusion at 1100 h*

* See later for glucose insulin infusions.
** Beware of patients on long acting sulphonylureas (e.g. glibenclamide). If they are on long acting tablets, consider stopping tablets in the morning.

- In the postoperative period, the diabetes team should be consulted about patients treated with sulphonylurea tablets, as they may need a phase of insulin treatment in the immediate postoperative period.

(iv) Patients on insulin therapy

Minor surgery – (No restrictions to eating in the postoperative period)

Morning list	Afternoon list
Fast from midnight	Fast from 0800 h
Glucose drink at 0600 h	Half morning dose of insulin
Delay insulin dose and breakfast until after procedure	Allow usual breakfast Glucose drink at 1030 h Delay lunchtime insulin and lunch until after procedure

■ If patient does not feel like a meal after the procedure, offer glucose drinks or snacks to avoid hypoglycaemia.

Major surgery – (Restrictions to eating in the immediate postoperative period)

Morning list	Afternoon list
Fast from midnight	Fast from 0800 h
No insulin in the morning	Half usual insulin dose before early breakfast
Start glucose insulin infusion at 0700 h	Start glucose insulin infusion at 1100 h

■ Consult diabetic team regarding return to subcutaneous regimen.

(v) Glucose-insulin infusions

■ In patients undergoing surgery, continuous intravenous insulin infusions generally attain better diabetes control and therefore reduced incidence of wound infection.

■ In critically ill patients, maintenance of plasma glucose between 4 and 6 mmol/l reduces morbidity and mortality.

There are two approaches to instituting a glucose-insulin regimen.

1. Intravenous dextrose with sliding scale insulin pump

■ Use 10% dextrose with 20 mmol KCl per litre and infuse intravenously, 1 litre per 8–12 h through an intravenous cannula. Make up an insulin syringe pump infusion by adding 50 units of soluble insulin (e.g. Actrapid®, Humulin S®) to 49 ml of 0.9% saline in a 50 ml syringe, which is infused through a separate cannula.

■ Measure capillary glucose by finger prick when commencing IV dextrose and insulin pump and hourly thereafter.

■ The insulin infusion rate is adjusted according to the capillary glucose. If the sliding scale insulin dosage fails to maintain adequate control (glucose ideally 4–7 mmol/l, adequate <10 mmol/l), alter the scale of insulin infusion to higher dose (see Table 11.1).

■ Remember – this regimen is intensive from the nursing perspective requiring hourly capillary glucose measurements and care needs to be taken to ensure IV dextrose and IV insulin run simultaneously. If one cannula becomes blocked or one infusion runs out, the patient may become hypoglycaemic or hyperglycaemic with potentially serious consequences.

11

Table 11.1 **Example of intravenous insulin pump sliding scale used with 10% dextrose IV infusion**

Blood glucose (mmol/l)	Insulin per hour (units)	Example of insulin dose adjustment if glucose levels too high (units)
<3.0	0	0
3.1–4.0	0.5	0.5
4.1–6.0	1	1
6.1–9.0	2	3
9.1–11.0	3	5
11.1–13.0	4	7
13.1–15.0	5	8
15.1–20.0	6	10
>20.0*	8	12

- Monitor capillary glucose hourly and adjust insulin dose accordingly.
- Check urea and electrolytes daily.
- Aim for glucose 4–7 mmol/l.
- Adjust insulin scale if glucose >10 mmol/l for >12 h.
- *If glucose >20 mmol/l, stop IV dextrose infusion, and switch to 0.9% saline.

- In some units, the insulin pump and the dextrose infusions go in through the same IV cannula (piggy back fashion), but it is essential that both infusions be mechanically driven.

2. GKI (Glucose Potassium Insulin) infusion

- To avoid some of the problems associated with the sliding scale insulin infusion, many centres now use the GKI (Glucose Potassium Insulin) infusion, which is simpler and ensures delivery of both glucose and insulin at an even rate.

- Use 10% dextrose 500 ml + 20 mmol (1.5 g) KCl + Actrapid insulin (dose per capillary glucose, see Table 11.2) to run over 6 h.

- Check blood glucose every 3 h and if insulin dose is not appropriate to achieve adequate diabetes control, start a new bag with the correct insulin dose.

- Exceptions to GKI

  1. Poorly Controlled Diabetes – achieve control of glucose with an insulin pump or multiple subcutaneous injections of rapid acting insulin and a basal intermediate insulin, prior to commencing the GKI infusion.

Table 11.2 **Example of GKI infusion regimen**

Blood glucose (mmol/l)	Actrapid insulin dose (units) in 10% dextrose 500 ml	Example of insulin dose adjustment if glucose levels too high
<2.9	0	0
3.0–5.9	5	5
6.0–9.9	10	10
10.0–13.9	15	20
14.0–19.9	20	30
>20.0	25	40

- Monitor capillary glucose 3-hourly and adjust insulin dose accordingly.
- Check urea and electrolytes daily.
- Aim for glucose 4–7 mmol/l.
- Adjust insulin scale if glucose >10 mmol/l for >12 h.

11

The Diabetes team will need to be consulted early for this to be effective.

2. Hyperkalaemia – omit the potassium in the infusion if K^+ is >5 mmol/l.

- Limitations of GKI

1. Dehydration – only provides 2 litres of fluid daily. Additional fluid may be required, but should not contain dextrose.

2. Hyponatraemia in prolonged infusions – avoid by giving IV 0.9% saline infusions at the same time.

3. Fluid balance in elderly and heart failure – If fluid restriction is needed, patients may need smaller volumes of 20% Dextrose to avoid fluid overload, e.g. the same amount of insulin and potassium in 250 ml of 20% dextrose over 12 h.

(vi) Changing from intravenous to subcutaneous insulin

- The $t_{1/2}$ of IV insulin is around 3 min.

- Insulin injected subcutaneously (even the so-called 'quick-acting' insulin analogues) takes at least 10–15 min for adequate levels to reach the bloodstream in order to control blood glucose.

- When an insulin-treated patient is eating and drinking, and is ready to go back onto their usual insulin regime, this should be done at a mealtime, with the subcutaneous insulin being given before the meal and the IV insulin infusion not to be stopped until 30 min after the meal.

Discharge of patient following surgery

- It is likely that glycaemic control will be disturbed for a time after discharge, although this depends on the severity of surgery and the convalescent period required.

- Most diabetic units have well trained diabetes nurse specialists who will be able to advise patients about managing their treatment to optimise glucose levels. The patients will often know who to contact in order to obtain this advice, which can be given over the telephone.

- If the diabetes nurse specialist has not been involved during the patient's hospital stay, they should be contacted prior to discharge so that appropriate follow up can be organised.

Further reading
1 Alberti KGMM, Gill GV and Elliott MJ. Insulin delivery during surgery in the diabetic patient. Diabetes Care 1982; 5:65–77.
2 Golden SH, Peart-Vigilance C, Kao WHL and Brancati FL. Perioperative glycemic control and the risk of infectious complications in a cohort of adults with diabetes. Diabetes Care 1999; 22:1408–1414.
3 Husband DJ, Thai AC and Alberti KGMM. Management of diabetes during surgery with glucose–insulin–potassium infusion. Diabetic Med 1986; 3:69–74.
4 Root HF. Preoperative care of the diabetic patient. Postgrad Med 1966; 40:439.
5 Berghe GV, Wouters P and Weekes F. Intensive insulin therapy in critically ill patients. N Engl J Med 2001; 345:1359–1367.

11

12

Causes and treatment of aspiration

Paul Hughes

Introduction

Normal breathing, speaking and swallowing are accompanied by efficient defence methods against aspiration of fluid and/or solids into the lower respiratory tract. Patients with impaired conscious levels, impaired cough and gag reflexes and susceptibility to regurgitation or vomiting are at risk of aspiration of gastric contents into the airway.

Pulmonary aspiration of gastric contents is one of the most feared complications of anaesthesia. It can lead to pneumonitis, pulmonary hypertension, ventilation-perfusion mismatch and acute respiratory distress syndrome (ARDS). Patients who have aspirated are eight times more likely to die after surgery. Prevention of aspiration forms the very basis of safe anaesthetic practice (see Chapter 6: Perioperative management of emergency surgery).

Precautions against aspiration include:

■ Identification of patients at risk.

■ Preoperative fasting.

■ Drug treatments, e.g. metoclopramide, H_2 antagonists, sodium citrate.

■ Anaesthetic techniques, e.g. rapid sequence induction with cricoid pressure.

Due to the care taken to avoid this complication in routine practice, the incidence of pulmonary aspiration in general surgical patients is small (<1 in 2,000) and only slightly greater in children and obstetric patients. Overall, morbidity is low and mortality is extremely rare (1 in 70,000 to 1 in 240,000 patients). There was one maternal death from pulmonary aspiration in 1991–1993.

Pathophysiology

In unconscious and anaesthetised patients, lower oesophageal tone decreases and laryngeal reflexes are depressed. Aspiration may follow passive regurgitation of gastric contents or vomiting, most commonly during induction of anaesthesia when the airway is unprotected.

Aspiration may present with acute airway obstruction if the aspirated matter is solid. More commonly it presents as gradual onset of respiratory distress and respiratory failure due to bacterial infection of the lungs or due to the inflammatory effects of acid aspiration. Up to one third of patients who aspirate will develop ARDS and this has a high mortality (40–60%) (Fig. 12.1).

History and examination

Acute aspiration usually presents with a history of vomiting or evidence of blood, vomitus or secretions in the mouth and airway. The patient usually

12

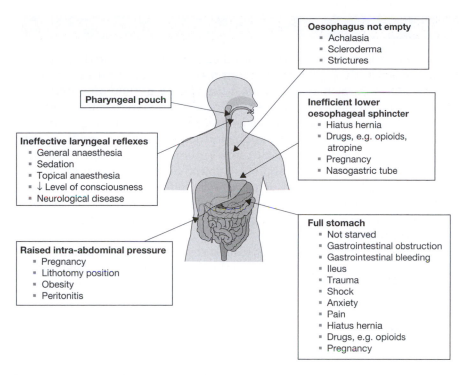

Oesophagus not empty
- Achalasia
- Scleroderma
- Strictures

Pharyngeal pouch

Inefficient lower oesophageal sphincter
- Hiatus hernia
- Drugs, e.g. opioids, atropine
- Pregnancy
- Nasogastric tube

Ineffective laryngeal reflexes
- General anaesthesia
- Sedation
- Topical anaesthesia
- ↓ Level of consciousness
- Neurological disease

Full stomach
- Not starved
- Gastrointestinal obstruction
- Gastrointestinal bleeding
- Ileus
- Trauma
- Shock
- Anxiety
- Pain
- Hiatus hernia
- Drugs, e.g. opioids
- Pregnancy

Raised intra-abdominal pressure
- Pregnancy
- Lithotomy position
- Obesity
- Peritonitis

Fig. 12.1 Factors predisposing to aspiration.

12

exhibits one or more of the risk factors listed above, and suddenly develops cough, dyspnoea, wheeze, tachypnoea, stridor, crepitations, rhonchi, cyanosis, hypotension, tachycardia and fever.

Chronic recurrent aspiration is usually seen in patients with neuromuscular disorders associated with disorders of bulbar function, and may present with a gradual deterioration of respiratory function and intermittent respiratory symptoms and signs. There may be a history of coughing or choking after food.

Acute aspiration of obstructive solids will lead to rapid hypoxaemia and death if the obstruction is not relieved. The patient will not be able to speak or breathe. Partial obstruction with smaller solids leads to varying degrees of the acute aspiration syndrome described above. If inhaled solids are not removed then secondary infection will occur leading to bacterial pneumonia, abscess formation and chronic infection (e.g. bronchiectasis).

Acid aspiration in large volumes produces a particular syndrome known as Mendelson's syndrome (C.L. Mendelson – U.S. obstetrician) characterised by severe dyspnoea, wheeze, hypoxaemia and shock. Acid secretions damage the alveolar lining of the lung, reduce surfactant, and lead to increased permeability with the development of pulmonary oedema and ARDS.

Investigations

In addition to the clinical features listed above which may be detected on physical examination, a full blood count may reveal leucocytosis with a left shift. Chest X-ray may be normal if the volume of fluid aspirated is small, or if taken early after the event. Focal consolidation is the most common finding and represents a chemical pneumonitis. Changes are commonly seen in the right upper lobe in supine aspiration and the right middle and lower lobes in sitting or semi-recumbent aspiration. Findings are bilateral in 70% of patients. Consolidation may progress rapidly to become a more diffuse process with diffuse infiltrates, collapse or severe pulmonary oedema. The radiological findings tend to worsen for several days then improve quickly, unless there is a superimposed bacterial pneumonia or ARDS.

Aspiration of particulate matter usually results in small, localised abnormalities due to collapse distal to the airway obstruction. Findings typically clear within 24–48 h, a mucociliary action and coughing clearing the airway. Persistent opacities suggest superimposed infection.

Other investigations that may assist in making the diagnosis include:

- Endotracheal suctioning to detect gastric contents or acidic pH on specific testing. All aspirates should be Gram-stained and cultured.

- Fibreoptic bronchoscopy to identify particulate matter.

- Clinical examination to detect laryngeal incompetence.

- Water soluble contrast (Omnipaque®) swallow in difficult diagnostic situations of recurrent aspiration.

Management

The Heimlich manoeuvre is indicated in complete airway obstruction (H.J. Heimlich – U.S. physician at Xavier University, Cincinnati, Ohio).

For lesser degrees of aspiration of gastric contents, management is as follows:

- The patient should be placed in the head-down right lateral position (this may localise aspiration to the right lung and prevent further aspiration).

- Material is aspirated from the pharynx and larynx.

- Oxygen is administered (humidified if possible).

- Clinical condition and oxygen saturation are monitored.

- Tracheal intubation may be necessary to protect the airway and to allow tracheobronchial suction.

12

- Antibiotics should be avoided unless there is evidence of infection. If required, therapy should be effective against the normal respiratory pathogens, Gram-negative organisms and anaerobic organisms.

- Bronchodilator therapy should be given to treat bronchospasm (e.g. inhaled β_2-adrenergic agents).

- A period of mechanical ventilatory support may be necessary in severe cases.

- Cardiovascular support may be necessary in the 'shock syndrome' associated with acid aspiration.

A rapid sequence induction and cricoid pressure (Sellick's manoeuvre) are often employed to attempt to prevent aspiration during the induction of anaesthesia (see Chapter 6: Perioperative management of emergency surgery).

Outcome

The clinical course of aspiration of non-acidic fluids is usually a rapidly resolving illness over a few days with few complications.

In infected, non-acid aspiration, the clinical course depends on the volume of aspirate, efficacy of antibiotics and whether lower respiratory infection becomes established. Initial hypoxia may be severe, but the shock and ARDS picture of acid aspiration are less common. The lung injury may gradually resolve or pneumonia may develop, leading to a more severe, protracted illness.

Acid aspiration precipitating ARDS is characterised by a severe pulmonary injury requiring prolonged mechanical ventilation and is often associated with sepsis and multiple organ failure. Mortality is high depending on the severity of aspiration and the presence of underlying disease states.

12

Key points

1. In the healthy individual aspiration of gastric contents is prevented by several physiological protective mechanisms in the upper gastrointestinal tract and upper airway.

2. Disease states and anaesthesia in healthy individuals can predispose an individual to aspiration.

3. Normal safe anaesthetic practice is directed towards preventing aspiration.

4. The consequences of aspiration range from sudden acute upper airway obstruction to subclinical progressive respiratory impairment in chronic disease states.

5. Aspiration associated with anaesthesia is usually clinically benign but in its most extreme form can lead to 'Mendelson's syndrome' associated with ARDS, sepsis syndrome and a high mortality.

6. The chest X-ray most commonly shows areas of focal consolidation, usually on the right side.

7. Treatment is directed towards preventing further contamination of the airway, administration of oxygen and monitoring respiratory function.

8. Further treatment may be required in more severe cases on an intensive care unit.

Further reading

Engelhardt T and Webster NR. Pulmonary aspiration of gastric contents in anaesthesia. Br J Anaesth 1999; 83:453–460.

Mendelson C. The aspiration of stomach contents into the lungs during obstetric anesthesia. Am J Obstet Gynecol 1946; 52:191–205.

12

13

Transfusion and blood products

Andy Johnston

Allogenic blood can be life saving, but it is a valuable and limited resource and has the potential for a number of adverse effects. This chapter will discuss the following aspects of blood transfusion

■ What is allogenic blood?

■ Who should blood be given to?

■ How should blood be given?

■ The adverse effects of blood transfusion.

What is allogenic blood?

A blood donor gives approximately 420 ml of blood and this is mixed with 70 ml of CAPD (citrate, adenine, phosphate and dextrose). Approximately 250 ml of plasma (with platelets) is removed and the red blood cells (RBCs) are resuspended in 100 ml of SAGM (saline, adenine, glucose and mannitol) to give approximately 300 ml of packed RBCs with a haematocrit (Hct) of 0.6–0.7. Since 1998 blood has been routinely depleted of leucocytes. The blood can be stored at 2–6°C for up to 35 days. These packed cells have a low pH, reduced 2,3-DPG (therefore a left shifted oxygen dissociation curve), high potassium (approximately 20 mmol/l after 20 days of storage), negligible viable platelets and reduced coagulation factors (especially V and VIII). After rewarming and transfusion the potassium is taken back up into RBCs and 2,3-DPG levels are normal by 24 h.

In a 70 kg adult, one unit of packed RBCs raises the haemoglobin concentration by approximately 1 g/dl.

Who should blood be given to?

Blood is required for oxygen delivery but the potential adverse effects of blood, the expense, and the fact that an increase in blood viscosity (with increasing haematocrit) may actually reduce oxygen delivery has meant that blood transfusion practice has become more restrictive in the last few years. A haemoglobin concentration of 7–8 g/dl is usually acceptable in the fit patient without ongoing blood loss or the potential for blood loss during surgery. Chronic anaemia is usually tolerated well in both fit and unfit patients, but anaemia with a short onset time is not tolerated well by patients with severe respiratory disease or ischaemic heart disease.

Fit patients with a Hb >7 g/dl should not be transfused routinely; when preoperative, such patients should be grouped and saved, or cross matched depending on the nature of the surgery. Unfit patients should be transfused up to a Hb >10 g/l and if this is being done preoperatively then ideally it should be more than 24 h before the operation (to allow restoration of RBC 2,3-DPG levels). Obviously, the unfit patient will still require a current group and save or cross match before surgery. The best advice is that each patient should be assessed individually and transfusion should be tailored to the individual.

For patients who are bleeding acutely, blood will be required if the patients are in class 3 shock (i.e. have lost 30–40% of their blood volume) or have other medical problems necessitating a more liberal policy. Pushing up the intravascular volume may make the bleeding worse so the priority is to stem the flow. Remember that packed cells have a haematocrit of 0.6–0.7 so ~500 ml of colloid should be given for every two units of red cells to give a normal haematocrit.

How to give blood

In an emergency situation O−ve blood (universal donor) can be given before a group and save (G + S) or cross match (X match) has been carried out. Group specific blood can be given following a G + S. These situations are unusual and blood is normally only given after a G + S and formal X match.

Transfusion of incompatible blood is most commonly due to human error and is a serious cause of morbidity and mortality. For these reasons, every step from the initial G + S to the eventual transfusion should be carried out meticulously.

The G + S sample will be used to determine the patient's blood group (ABO and Rhesus), may be screened to determine atypical antibodies against other groups and will eventually be used for cross matching purposes. It is therefore vital that the G + S sample is taken from the correct patient and labelled correctly. The patient's identity band should accurately match the notes and the name, date of birth (DOB) and hospital number should match that written on the blood bottle and on the transfusion laboratory request form. The transfusion laboratory requires at least three identity categories (normally name, DOB and hospital number) and will automatically reject any incomplete or illegible requests, or any incompletely filled sample bottles.

Once a G + S has been performed, the laboratory is able to X match blood by adding recipient serum to RBCs from each donor unit. Agglutination, after incubation for 30–60 min, means that the recipient has antibodies against donor RBC antigens and thus, that unit of donor blood is incompatible. Once blood has been X matched, it is issued by the laboratory and is available for transfusion.

When X matched blood is required for transfusion it is collected from the fridge by a trained member of staff, as and when needed. If too much is collected it will warm up to room temperature and become unusable after a few hours. A temperature sensitive label on the unit of blood will indicate this has happened.

Before the blood is given it must be thoroughly checked. Both the blood and the transfusion slip which accompanies it must be checked against both the patient's identity band and the patient's notes and ALL the details must match. The blood unit number, blood group and expiry

13

date must exactly match the details on the transfusion slip. It is only when all these details have been checked by at least two trained members of staff that the blood can be transfused.

The blood is transfused via a blood giving set which contains a filter removing fibrin aggregates and RBC aggregates. The speed of transfusion will depend on the clinical circumstances, but if not being used to replace acute blood loss, then 2–4 h per unit is usually adequate. If the patient has a low Hct/Hb but is normovolaemic then colloid/crystalloid is not required to correct for the high haematocrit of the packed cells. If the patient is at risk of cardiac failure from the increase in circulating blood volume then the transfusion should be slow and furosemide (frusemide) (20–40 mg PO/IV) is often given with every other unit.

The risk of adverse events requires that the patient be closely monitored during transfusion.

Adverse effects

Transfusion reactions

■ The most important is the haemolytic transfusion reaction, which is caused by recipient antibodies directed against donor cell antigens. ABO incompatibility, due to clerical errors, is the most frequent cause (risk ~0.6%). Features include rapid onset of fever, joint and back pain, skin rash, cardiovascular collapse and dyspnoea. DIC and renal failure may occur. Immediate management is to stop the transfusion and to resuscitate the patient as for an anaphylactic reaction. This will involve respiratory support (oxygen initially), volume resuscitation and adrenaline (epinephrine) (boluses of 0.1 mg IV). Immediate senior support is indicated. Samples of recipient and donor blood should urgently be sent to the transfusion laboratory.

■ Recipient antibodies to Rh or non-ABO blood types cause delayed extravascular haemolysis. This usually occurs 7–10 days post transfusion with fever, anaemia and jaundice. Renal failure may occur.

■ Non-haemolytic febrile reactions are due to recipient antibodies against donor leucocytes or platelets. There is usually slow onset of fever, dyspnoea and tachycardia; shock is rare. The transfusion should be stopped and the advice of a haematologist should be sought. Minor reactions can usually be treated by slowing the infusion rate and giving paracetamol and/or steroids.

■ Anaphylactoid reactions are a result of proteins in the donor plasma causing minor allergic reactions. They can usually be treated with antihistamines or steroids but haematological advice should be obtained.

■ True anaphylactic reactions may rarely occur.

13

Immunomodulation

The incidence of postoperative infections is elevated in transfused patients and cancer recurrence may be increased.

Exposure to donor antigens may make cross matching/tissue typing increasingly difficult in the future.

Transmission of infectious diseases

The risk of transmission of hepatitis B or C is ~1 in 30,000, for HIV it is ~1 in 1,000,000. Human T cell leukaemia and lymphoma virus (HTLV-1) may be transmitted, which is not screened for in the UK. Malaria, syphilis, cytomegalovirus, glandular fever and brucellosis may all be transmitted. Hepatitis G virus, variant Creutzfeld-Jakob disease and as yet unknown pathogens may all cause problems in the future. Rarely, bacterial contamination of donor units may cause fever and cardiovascular collapse.

Pulmonary dysfunction

Transfusion related acute lung injury may result from platelet micro aggregates or donor antibodies against recipient antigens.

Massive transfusion

One definition of massive transfusion is replacement of the patient's entire blood volume with transfused blood within 24 h. Massive transfusion may cause a number of problems.

- Hyperkalaemia and acidosis.

- Citrate toxicity may cause hypocalcaemia.

- Hypothermia. All transfused blood should be warmed, especially when infused rapidly.

- Impaired coagulation (rarely DIC). The coagulopathy associated with massive blood transfusion should normally be treated using laboratory clotting tests as a guide. FFP, platelets and cryoprecipitate may all be needed. Advice to give fresh frozen plasma (FFP) with every 4th unit of blood is now outdated.

- Impaired oxygen delivery to tissues.

Strategies for avoiding blood transfusion

- no operation

- good haemostasis

- autologous transfusion (2–6 units may be donated up to 6 weeks preoperatively)

- tourniquet, if surgery is to an extremity

- controlled hypotension

13

- isovolaemic transfusion

- hypervolaemic transfusion

- cell saver

- maximise oxygen delivery

- erythropoietin

- artificial 'blood'

Artificial 'blood'

These are man-made solutions capable of gas transport and oxygen delivery to tissues. There is a great deal of interest in these solutions since their utilisation avoids the risks of blood transfusion and there is no need for cross matching. Currently there are three groups:

- perfluorocarbons   e.g. Fluosol-DA (able to carry more oxygen than plasma, but side effects and short half-life have limited its use)

- recombinant Hb   (produced from *E. coli* and cleared by the reticulo-endothelial system)

- purified Hb   (salvaged from expired red cells)

Key points

- Blood products are expensive and a limited resource.

- Think carefully about the need for blood; some patients may be better off without it.

- Double check every step involved with blood transfusion.

- Be aware of potential adverse effects and how to manage them.

- Liaise closely with the transfusion laboratory.

- Always ask for help if you need it.

Further reading

The risks and uses of donated blood. Drug Ther Bull 1993; 31(23):89–92.

14

The critically ill patient

Vilas Navapurkar

Introduction

Critically ill patients are those who:

■ require or are likely to require respiratory support alone, or

■ require the support of two or more organ systems, or

■ have chronic impairment of one or more organ systems sufficient to restrict daily activities (comorbidity) and require support for an acute reversible failure of another organ system(s)

Such patients need to be cared for in an intensive care unit (ICU) which provides a *'service for patients with potentially recoverable conditions who can benefit from more detailed observation and invasive treatment than can safely be provided in general wards or high dependency areas'*. Those patients admitted to ICU from the hospital ward tend to have a higher mortality than those admitted from other hospital areas such as the accident and emergency department, even though they have, on occasion, been on the ward for several days. A proactive approach to the early identification of patients with or at risk of a critical illness may allow treatment to be instituted before irreversible single or multiple organ dysfunction is established and thus prevent mortality or limit morbidity.

Diagnosis of the critically ill patient

Patients usually develop (and die from) critical illnesses in predictable and reproducible patterns. Therefore, medical and nursing staff need to identify those at risk early and monitor their condition carefully.

Patients at risk of critical illness

Several groups of patients are at increased risk of becoming critically ill due to the nature of the presenting disease(s), insufficient physiological reserve to cope with an illness or, unfortunately, due to sub-optimal care. These patients need to be carefully observed for evidence of clinical deterioration and immediate and appropriate action taken to halt their decline (Table 14.1).

Antecedents and signs of critical illness

Before admission to ICU most patients have documented physiological dysfunction that often progresses to the need for cardiopulmonary resuscitation. The primary pathophysiological abnormalities before cardiac arrest are respiratory, metabolic, cardiac and neurological and these are usually interlinked. Clinical antecedents based on physiological criteria have been identified to produce ward based protocols or scoring systems to diagnose impending or established critical illness. An example is the Cambridge ICU Outreach 'Modified Early Warning Score' (MEWS) (Table 14.2).

14

Table 14.1 Patients at risk of critical illness

- emergencies
- elderly
- significant comorbidity, e.g. cardiorespiratory disease
- major surgery/trauma
- minor surgery in patients with significant comorbidity
- massive transfusion
- shock states, e.g. septic shock, cardiogenic shock

Patients exposed to poor practise:

- incomplete/infrequent assessment
- failure to act on abnormal findings
- inadequate basic support (e.g. oxygen therapy, hydration, analgesia, physiotherapy)
- failure to seek senior advice

Most patients present with multi-system dysfunction and it is sometimes difficult to identify the causative pathology. However, once a patient is thought to have an impending or established critical illness, early liaison with 'patient at risk teams' (PART) or ICU 'Outreach' teams has been shown to reduce both morbidity and mortality.

Initial management of the critically ill patient

Although the initial management can be subdivided, as below, the individual processes often occur simultaneously to form a continuum of care from the ward, operating theatre or accident and emergency department. Suggested subdivisions are:

- immediate management
- full assessment
- transfer to ICU
- initial care on ICU
- care of the ICU patient's family

Immediate assessment

An awareness of the relative importance of individual clinical signs is crucial. For example, an obstructed airway will kill more quickly than

14

Table 14.2 The Cambridge ICU Outreach Modified Early Warning Score (MEWS)

Score	3	2	1	0	1	2	3
HR (beats/min)		<40	42–50	51–100	101–110	111–129	>130
RR (breaths/min)		<8		9–14	15–20	21–29	>30
Systolic BP (mmHg)	<70	71–80	81–100	109–180		>180	
CNS GCS	Unresponsive	Pain	Voice	Alert 15	Confused 14	9–13	≤8
Urine output	Nil	<1 ml/kg for 2 h	<1 ml/kg/h				>400 ml/h
Temp (°C)		<35		35–38.4		38.5–39	>39

CNS = Central nervous system, GCS = Glasgow Coma Scale.

When to use
Any patient you are worried about, even if that judgement is based on instinct (never underestimate instinct!).

When to contact Outreach team
Formal referral if score 4 or >4.

Informal referral
If support or advice is required (e.g. help setting up CVP) or score is <4 but you are still concerned.

cardiac dysfunction. Therefore, the aim of the *immediate* assessment is the *immediate* treatment of life threatening problems.

A – Airway
Signs of a compromised airway are:

■ absent or low frequency (<8 breaths/min) respiratory effort

■ tracheal tug, 'see-saw' breathing pattern, abdominal breathing and an impaired level of consciousness all imply an obstructed airway as does stridor and the inability to feel airflow from the mouth or nose

High flow oxygen (12–15 l/min by a rebreathing bag) should be given immediately once the airway has been cleared and maintained. This can be achieved by a jaw thrust, suction of debris or vomitus, the insertion of a

Guedel airway and ultimately the insertion of a cuffed endotracheal tube by an anaesthetist.

B – Breathing

Inadequate ventilation can be inferred from:

- rapid, shallow breathing

- cyanosis

- the use of accessory muscles or paradoxical abdominal movement

- inability to talk or complete sentences

- tracheal deviation, surgical emphysema

The precise treatment will depend on the cause of inadequate ventilation. If inadequate ventilation is due to tension pneumothorax, which is life-threatening, it should be treated immediately with a wide bore cannula placed in to the pleural cavity on the side of the pneumothorax in the second intercostal space in the mid-axillary line, followed by formal placement of an intercostal chest drain connected to an underwater seal.

C – Circulation

Hypovolaemia should always be considered the primary problem in circulatory failure in most critically ill patients and a bolus of fluid (10–20 ml/kg) should be given. Closer monitoring and a lower fluid dose (5 ml/kg) should be given if congestive cardiac failure is the most likely cause. Blood pressure can be normal in a shocked patient especially if they are young. Signs of inadequate peripheral perfusion (pallor, coolness, underfilled veins), obvious haemorrhage and a rapid, thready pulse are all suggestive of circulatory compromise. Rarely, it is necessary to commence an adrenaline infusion immediately to try to establish a blood pressure safe enough to transport a critically ill patient to the ICU.

D – Dysfunction of the CNS

A rapid assessment of the patient's neurological status can be made using the Glasgow Coma Scale. Patients with a GCS ≤8 are likely to have lost protective airway reflexes and require endotracheal intubation to avoid aspiration of gastric contents or upper airway secretions.

14

E – Exposure

A comprehensive assessment can only be made by examining the adequately exposed patient. Care must be taken to prevent hypothermia and to ensure that the patient's dignity is maintained at all times.

Throughout each of these stages the patient should be constantly reassessed to monitor their response to treatment. A failure to respond or a temporary or inadequate response means that different treatment and senior help is required immediately.

Full assessment

A full assessment of the patient's history with particular reference to comorbidity and current medication should be conducted as soon as practicable. The patient should also be examined thoroughly and the value of repeated clinical examination to monitor treatment and elicit signs should not be underestimated. A systematic review of the charts, notes, investigations and results will provide crucial data about the patient's condition, rate of decline and physiological reserve.

Transfer to ICU

The primary goals of safely transferring a critically ill patient are:

■ physiological stability

■ adequate ventilation

■ secure intravenous access

■ appropriate monitoring

■ communication with the nursing staff and the patient's family

Careful patient preparation by doctors experienced in resuscitation and organ support will reduce the risks of complications during transfer. A patent and protected airway together with adequate ventilation and secure intravenous access must be guaranteed before moving a patient. This often requires sedation, analgesia and even muscle paralysis if controlled ventilation is required. Monitoring of the patient should be as comprehensive as is feasible but should always include a continuous electrocardiogram, intermittent non-invasive blood pressure measurement and pulse oximetry. Institution of invasive blood pressure monitoring is advisable if the patient requires transfer to another hospital. Early communication with the ICU staff and details of the patient's immediate requirements will allow them time to prepare the necessary equipment and infusions thus preventing delays in treatment. It is also imperative to explain as much as possible to the patient's family to help them cope during this extremely stressful and frightening time.

Initial care on the ICU

Due to the complexity of illnesses in ICU patients, a systematic and multi-disciplinary approach to the assessment, support and monitoring of each organ system will allow a coherent treatment strategy for organ support to be developed. Most patients will need multiple lumen central venous access, continuous intra-arterial blood pressure monitoring, hourly urine volume measurement and at least intermittent core temperature assessment in addition to the basic monitoring already established. Immediate changes to treatment can be guided by early analysis of the arterial blood gases. If the patient's condition deteriorates or more data about his/her condition is required then further invasive monitors, such as a pulmonary artery catheter, may be used.

14

a. Sedation and analgesia

Patients require sedation and analgesia to reduce pain and anxiety, tolerate medical and nursing procedures, allow adequate ventilation and to help maintain cardiovascular stability. Combinations of drugs, either as infusions or bolus doses, are used (usually administered via a central vein). Commonly used drugs are:

- intravenous anaesthetic agents (propofol, thiopentone, ketamine)
- benzodiazepines (midazolam, lorazepam, diazepam, temazepam)
- opioids (remifentanil, alfentanil, fentanyl, morphine, pethidine)
- others (NSAIDs, isoflurane, phenothiazines, chlormethiazole)

b. Ventilation

There is a variety of ventilatory patterns employed depending on the nature of the patient's illness and it is the ventilatory requirement that is the main determinant of how deeply a patient is sedated. Frequent arterial blood gas measurements are used to monitor the efficiency of gas exchange and the P_aO_2 should generally be maintained at 8.5 kPa or higher. Some patients may be difficult to oxygenate and require muscle paralysis or ventilation in the prone position.

ARDS (adult respiratory distress syndrome) can be defined as diffuse pulmonary infiltrates (on CXR), refractory hypoxaemia, stiff lungs and respiratory distress following a recognised precipitating cause. Some definitions include the ratio of the partial pressure of oxygen in arterial blood to the fraction of inspired oxygen (P_aO_2/F_iO_2). A pulmonary artery occlusion pressure of <16 mmHg is generally included in the definition, in order to exclude cardiogenic causes. Trauma, shock, sepsis, massive blood transfusion, pulmonary aspiration, pneumonia, pancreatitis and amniotic fluid embolism have all been associated with ARDS.

c. Cardiovascular support

Signs of inadequate tissue perfusion are:

- arterial hypotension (systolic less than 90 mmHg)
- oliguria (<0.5 ml/kg/h)
- confusion, agitation or decreased concious level
- cold, clammy, mottled skin
- metabolic acidaemia (base deficiency more than −4 mmol/l) and a raised serum lactate (>2 mmol/l)

14

The causes are hypovolaemia, cardiogenic shock (commonly post myocardial infarction), septic shock and combinations of all three. The primary treatment aims are to establish normovolaemia, a haemoglobin concentration of at least 8.5 g/dl and the use of inotropes either to increase the cardiac output and/or the systemic vascular resistance and hopefully reverse the consequences of tissue hypoperfusion. Commonly used inotropes are adrenaline (epinephrine), noradrenaline (norepinephrine), dopamine, dobutamine and dopexamine (see Chapter 15: Inotropes). If the patients have sepsis or are persistently hypovolaemic, supportive measures will only temporise unless the underlying condition is treated.

SIRS (systemic inflammatory response syndrome) is the response to many severe clinical insults and is manifested by two or more of the following:

- Temperature >38°C or <36°C

- Heart rate >90 beats/min

- Respiratory rate >20 breaths/min (or $PaCO_2$ <4.3 kPa)

- White cell count >12,000 cells/mm^3 or <4,000 cells/mm^3

There are many different disease processes involved in SIRS, but all are thought to involve activation of the cytokine cascade.

Sepsis is defined as SIRS occurring as a result of documented infection. Severe sepsis generally implies organ dysfunction and hypoperfusion or hypotension as a result of infection. Severe sepsis is directly or indirectly implicated in up to 75% of deaths in intensive care.

d. Other measures

Patients may also require urgent renal replacement therapy in the form of continuous veno-venous haemofiltration (CVVHF) if they have acute renal failure and are hyperkalaemic and/or fluid overloaded. Furthermore, hypothermia and hyperthermia should both be prevented or corrected although there is some evidence that moderate hypothermia may improve outcome in some groups of patients. Risk factors for the development of gastric stress ulceration and consequent haemorrhage are sepsis, hypovolaemia, burns, trauma and mechanical ventilation. Protective strategies should be started early on and usually consist of ensuring adequate tissue oxygen delivery and the use of sucralfate to line and protect the gastric mucosa. Some patients such as those with gastrointestinal bleeding or those on high dose steroids will also benefit from the use of proton pump inhibitors such as pantoprazole. Assuming the patient does not have a coagulopathy he/she is at increase risk of deep venous thrombosis and therefore pulmonary thromboembolism. Prophylaxis with low molecular weight heparin, whilst ensuring adequate hydration, should be started as soon as possible. Antibiotics are widely used in the ICU but they should, as much as possible, be guided by microbiological screening and sensitivity results.

Care of the ICU patient's family

An admission to ICU is frightening for the patient's family and there is a significant risk that the patient may die depending on the nature of the illness, physiological reserve and the response to treatment. It is important

14

to be clear and honest with the family and avoid comforting them with possibly unrealistic hopes. However, all discussions should be as empathic and as compassionate as possible and be clearly documented and witnessed in the medical and nursing notes.

A patient's chance of surviving a critical illness is greatly enhanced by prompt identification, rapid adequate treatment and the early involvement of the appropriate medical and nursing staff. Clearly prevention is always to be favoured and the early identification of those at risk together with close surveillance is crucial.

Key points

■ prompt and rapid diagnosis of critically ill patients is essential for a good outcome

■ 'early warning scores' can help all staff to recognise/predict critical illness

■ initial aims are the immediate treatment of life threatening problems

■ not all critically ill patients will benefit from critical care services (especially those who are terminally ill or have little prospect of recovery)

Further reading

1 Guidelines on Admission to and Discharge from Intensive Care and High Dependency Units. Department of Health, March 1996.
2 McQuillan P, Pilkington S, Allan A, Taylor B, Short A, Morgan G, et al. Confidential inquiry into quality of care before admission to intensive care. BMJ 1998; 316:1853–1858.
3 Goldhill DR, Worthington L, Mulcahy A, Tarling M and Sumner A. The patient-at-risk team: identifying and managing seriously ill ward patients. Anaesthesia 1999; 54:853–860.

14

15

Inotropes

Andy Gregg

Introduction

An inotrope is a drug that increases the force of myocardial contraction. This improves cardiac output, which raises blood flow and oxygen delivery to vital organs. Increased myocardial contractility unfortunately requires greater myocardial oxygen consumption.

Inotropes will move the Frank-Starling curve upwards (as shown in Figure 15.1), from line A to line B, such that for a given filling pressure of the heart, the cardiac output is increased. However the greatest effect is when the heart is optimally volume filled at position X (arrowed).

Sympathomimetics

These inotropes act directly on alpha and beta adrenoreceptors, but unfortunately none are completely selective. A summary of the major adrenoreceptor locations and their effects is shown in Table 15.1.

Endogenous catecholamines

Dopamine stimulates beta-receptors at lower doses (2–$10\,\mu g\,kg^{-1}min^{-1}$), but as the dose increases beyond $10\,\mu g\,kg^{-1}min^{-1}$, alpha effects predominate. There are also specific dopamine receptors that cause renal and splanchnic vessel dilatation, however clinically there is no evidence that stimulating these provides any benefit in preventing renal dysfunction.

Adrenaline (Epinephrine) is synthesised from noradrenaline (norepinephrine) and stimulates both alpha and beta-receptors resulting in inotropy, chronotropy and vasoconstriction.

Noradrenaline (Norepinephrine) is synthesised from dopamine and although it stimulates alpha and beta-receptors, noradrenaline

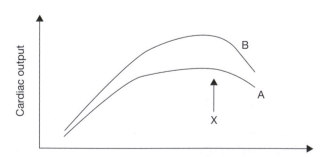

Filling pressure (CVP) or end diastolic volume of the heart

Fig. 15.1 Graph showing the relationship between cardiac output and filling pressure; a modification of the Frank-Starling curve which plotted the force of cardiac myocyte contraction against initial fibre length.

Table 15.1 **The location of adrenoreceptors and physiological effects of their stimulation**

Adrenoreceptor	Location	Effect of stimulation
Alpha-1	Vascular smooth muscle	Vasoconstriction
Beta-1	Heart	Increased heart rate (chronotropy) and myocardial contractility (inotropy)
Beta-2	Vascular smooth muscle	Vasodilatation

(norepinephrine) has a far greater alpha effect than adrenaline (epinephrine) at equivalent doses.

Synthetic agents

Dobutamine acts on beta-1 receptors causing inotropy and chronotropy, but also has a beta-2 effect that results in systemic vasodilatation.

Dopexamine is a beta-2 agonist, but does not have any alpha or beta-1 effects. It also stimulates peripheral dopaminergic receptors. The use of dopexamine to specifically increase renal and splanchnic blood flow is controversial.

Ephedrine displaces noradrenaline (norepinephrine) from sympathetic nerve endings into the synaptic cleft causing a non-selective sympathetic effect. Repeated administration will deplete presynaptic noradrenaline (norepinephrine) stores, reducing efficacy. Ephedrine also stimulates alpha and beta adrenoreceptors directly.

Phenylephrine and metaraminol both exhibit effects similar to noradrenaline (norepinephrine). Ephedrine, phenylephrine and metaraminol tend to be used during operations, in occasional bolus doses, if a transient need for an inotrope arises.

Other inotropes

Phosphodiesterase inhibitors

Stimulated beta adrenoreceptors activate adenyl cyclase intracellularly, which produces the secondary messenger cyclic adenosine monophosphate (cAMP). The cAMP then causes the biological effects such as increased inotropy via a number of mechanisms. cAMP is metabolised by phosphodiesterase enzymes. Inhibition of these enzymes will result in prolongation of increased levels of cAMP causing an increased biological effect. There are five isoenzymes of phosphodiesterase located in different tissues.

15

Aminophylline is a non-specific phosphodiesterase inhibitor, producing widespread effects throughout many organ systems, and usually used as a bronchodilator.

Milrinone and enoximone are selective inhibitors of phosphodiesterase isoenzyme (III) located in the heart and vascular smooth muscle. They cause inotropy and vasodilatation.

Drugs increasing intracellular calcium

Calcium binds to tropomyosin and increases cross bridging with actin, causing myofilament excitation-contraction coupling. The strength of contraction improves when more calcium binding sites are occupied on tropomyosin.

Digoxin is commonly used to control the rate of fast atrial fibrillation, but has a weak inotropic action as it inhibits membrane-bound $Na^+/K^+/ATPase$ enzymes. This inhibition causes a rise in intracellular sodium and calcium. Digoxin is the only inotrope that does not cause a tachycardia.

Glucagon causes an increase in production of cAMP, which results in increased intracellular calcium. This is classically quoted as the inotrope of choice in beta-blocker overdose.

Calcium given intravenously will have an inotropic effect, particularly in hypocalcaemic patients.

Practical application

Inotropes are mostly used to improve the function of a failing heart pump, or to assist a heart in the presence of severe sepsis. In both states inotropes may be indicated if there is evidence of poor organ perfusion. This may be clinically identified by confusion from poor cerebral perfusion, low urine output from poor renal perfusion, or cool peripheries from poor skin perfusion. It is important to remember that the target is organ perfusion and not blood pressure. This is because the wrong inotrope can temporarily create a normal blood pressure due to excessive vasoconstriction in the presence of a low cardiac output. The result would be further reduction of organ perfusion.

Before inotropes are started, the heart should be optimally volume filled. This is essential, because optimal left ventricular filling will maximise cardiac output (as can be seen from the Frank-Starling curve in Figure 15.1), and so may negate or reduce inotrope requirement. Optimal volume filling can be difficult to determine, but poor skin turgor and a dry mouth suggest an under-filled cardiovascular system. A raised jugular venous pressure, the presence of a third heart sound and pulmonary oedema would suggest a fluid overloaded cardiovascular system. Further evidence of volume status can be gained from measurement of central venous pressure, or pulmonary artery occlusion pressure.

Inotropes should be used in minimal doses required to achieve adequate organ perfusion, as they have side effects of tachycardia, arrhythmias, hyperglycaemia and increased myocardial oxygen consumption. Dobutamine, dopexamine and the catecholamines have short plasma half-lives of only a few minutes and are therefore given as intravenous infusions. These infusions will cause skin necrosis if they extravasate and should ideally be given via a central venous catheter. Because of their high potency and side effects, they should be used in closely observed and monitored locations, such as high dependency units (HDU), intensive care units (ICU) and operating theatres. Ideally, continuous invasive blood pressure monitoring should be employed. An exception to all of this is the emergency use of 1 mg of adrenaline (epinephrine) as an intravenous bolus (10 ml of 1 in 10,000) in cardiac arrest, or an intra-muscular injection (1 ml of 1 in 1,000) in anaphylaxis.

Choice of inotrope

Which inotrope to use in a given clinical situation is a matter of opinion. Generally however, dopamine or adrenaline (epinephrine) is used primarily to increase cardiac output. They may require addition of a vasodilator to counteract the vasoconstriction seen as the dose increases. Noradrenaline (norepinephrine) is the usual inotrope of choice in severe sepsis, as its vasoconstriction counteracts the endotoxin-induced vasodilatation. Dobutamine or a phosphodiesterase III inhibitor is used in primary cardiogenic failure with high afterload, as they also cause some vasodilatation.

Following optimal volume filling, if poor organ perfusion persists, there can still be a question as to relative degree of cardiogenic failure, vasodilatation or vasoconstriction. An assessment of cardiac output and systemic vascular resistance should then be made using a pulmonary artery catheter, an oesophageal doppler probe or a lithium dilutional technique. The results will then help guide the choice of inotrope, based on which physiological parameter should be manipulated, and in which direction.

Key points

■ Inotropes increase the force of myocardial contraction and thereby improve cardiac output, but increase myocardial oxygen demand.

■ Optimal volume filling should precede use of inotropes.

■ Noradrenaline (norepinephrine) is a vasoconstrictor.

■ Patients receiving inotropes should be managed on a critical care unit.

■ Cardiac output and systemic vascular resistance assessment can help guide the choice of inotrope when clinical uncertainty exists.

15

Further reading

Bellomo R, Chapman M, Finfer S, Hickling K and Myburgh J. Low-dose dopamine in patients with early renal dysfunction: a placebo-controlled randomised trial. Lancet 2000; 356:2139–2143.

Drugs and the autonomic system. In: Calvey TN and Williams NE. Principles and Practice of Pharmacology for Anaesthetists. Blackwell Science, Oxford 1997, pp 414–447.

Takala J, Meier-Hellmann A, Eddleston J, Hulstaert P and Sramek V. Effect of dopexamine on outcome after major abdominal surgery: a prospective randomised, controlled multicenter study. Critical Care Medicine 2000; 28:3417–3423.

16

Arterial blood gases

Simon Fletcher

16

The sampling of arterial blood for analysis of *blood gases* and *acid-base status* is now a routine part of the assessment of acutely ill patients and also part of the preoperative work up in an increasing number.

It is an invaluable monitoring tool in the critically ill, changes over both the short and intermediate term being indicative of a patient's response to therapeutic interventions.

Modern, rapid and accurate bench top analysers have both allowed and facilitated this. Many of these devices also measure single ion concentration as well as blood lactate, glucose and other simple parameters.

Blood gases analysis is an invaluable aid to the diagnosis, assessment of severity of physiological derangements and monitoring of the effectiveness of an intervention. Blood gases should never be interpreted in isolation, being part of the overall patient assessment.

Reproduced in Table 16.1 is a sample of a blood gas analysis, the read out customised to local requirements. When discussing the interpretation of blood gases, reference to this should help to understand the relevant principles.

When taking or interpreting blood gases the following must always be considered.

i. The analyser must be regularly calibrated to ensure accuracy of results.

ii. Use lightly heparinised blood samples to prevent costly blockage of the microcapillary tubes in an analyser. Excess heparin may give an erroneously low pH.

iii. Individuals should be appropriately trained on arterial blood gas (ABG) analyser usage.

iv. Avoid undue delay before analysis as red blood cells continue to metabolise in the interim.

v. Avoid excessive exposure of the sample to air.

vi. Note the fraction of inspired oxygen (F_IO_2) and temperature of the patient, so that these can be entered into the analyser.

The principles underlying the measurement of the various parameters will not be discussed except to say that pO_2, pH and pCO_2 are directly measured while many other factors are mathematically derived, some with the aid of 'correction factors'.

Assessment of the adequacy of ventilation/gas exchange

Ventilation

The arterial carbon dioxide partial pressure (P_aCO_2) is the most sensitive to changes in alveolar minute ventilation and in health should be around

16

Table 16.1 **Arterial blood gas analysis**

ABL725 ITU2 Patient report	Syringe – S 95 ul	Normal ranges
Identifications		
Patient ID	i8	
Operator	anniew	
Sample type	Arterial	
F_IO_2	60.0%	
Temp	37°C	
Blood gas values		
pH	7.214	7.35–7.45
cH_c^+	61.1 nmol/l	35–45 nmol/l
pCO_2	6.14 kPa	4.5–6.0 kPa
pO_2	11.6 kPa	11–14 kPa
Oximetry values		
ctHb	10.5 g/dl	
sO_2	97.6%	
Electrolyte values		
cK^+	3.6 mmol/l	3.5–5.0 mmol/l
cNa^+	135 mmol/l	135–145 mmol/l
Metabolite values		
cGlu	9.2 mmol/l	4.0–7.0 mmol/l
cLac	1.3 mmol/l	0.6–1.8 mmol/l
Acid base status		
$cBase(Ecf)_c$	−8.5 mmol/l	−2.0–+2.0 mmol/l
$cHCO_3^-(P,st)_c$	17.1 mmol/l	21–25 mmol/l

5.3 kPa. Some patients with chronic respiratory disease may normally have an elevated P_aco_2 and it is this group that rely on hypoxic drive to stimulate their ventilation. Typically, such a patient will have advanced chronic respiratory disease.

CO$_2$ reacts with water in blood to produce bicarbonate (HCO_3^-) and hydrogen (H^+) ions. Bicarbonate is the most important extracellular buffer and it is apparent therefore that changes in CO_2 are inexorably linked to acid/base status. Thus an 'abnormal' CO_2 concentration may actually be secondary to a primary metabolic disorder. This will be discussed in more detail below.

Oxygenation

The arterial O$_2$ tension (P_aO_2) is a measure of the adequacy of gas exchange. In health this is normally around 13.5 kPa, breathing room air.

16

Because of the shape of the O_2-haemoglobin dissociation curve, a P_aO_2 of greater than 8 kPa is often regarded as adequate. Haemoglobin saturation is approximately 90% at this level.

Interpretation of P_aO_2

Knowing this figure in isolation is of limited use. There are two major considerations:

1. Is the gas exchange process significantly deranged?

Referring to our reproduced blood gases, the patient has an adequate P_aO_2 of 11.6 kPa and would appear to have little wrong with his/her gas exchange. This would be true if the gases had been measured breathing room air (21% oxygen), but in fact they were taken on 60% oxygen. Thus a P_aO_2 must always be considered with the associated inspired oxygen concentration (F_IO_2).

Numerically, there is a way of relating these two figures: the P_aO_2/F_IO_2 ratio. The F_IO_2 is the 'fraction of inspired O_2', in this case 0.6: thus P_aO_2/F_IO_2 ratio is approximately 17, the normal being about 65. This patient, by definition therefore has severe acute lung injury (P_aO_2/F_IO_2 ratio <27).

There are numerous causes of deranged gas exchange but they essentially fall into two groups:

Non pulmonary
Hypoventilation (which will always be associated with a high P_aCO_2)
Low cardiac output states (in this case hypoxia is often associated with a low P_aCO_2)
Intra pulmonary (lung disease), essentially leading to ventilation/perfusion mismatch

2. There is a very important further consideration – is adequate P_aO_2 complimented by adequate tissue oxygenation?

The vast majority of oxygen is carried attached to haemoglobin and thus even with a normal P_aO_2, patients with low haemoglobin will have much reduced blood oxygen carriage. Other compounds also attach to haemoglobin, some with a greater affinity than oxygen. Carbon monoxide for instance has 200 times the affinity for haemoglobin than oxygen and thus even a moderately elevated level will reduce the amount of haemoglobin available to carry oxygen.

Even if arterial oxygen content is reasonable, adequate delivery also depends on blood flow and this may be globally or regionally abnormal for a multitude of reasons.

Inadequate tissue oxygenation will lead to a disturbance in acid/base status. How this may present, and other patterns of acid base abnormality are discussed below.

Acid-base balance

A straightforward, and in most circumstances reliable way of interpreting acid-base status involves the indices derived from the Henderson-Hasselbach (H-H) approach to the CO_2 – carbonic acid – HCO_3^- equilibrium. The relevant equation is:

$$pH = pK_a + \log_{10} [HCO_3^-]/PCO_2 \times 0.23 \text{ (solubility coefficient of } CO_2)$$

pH and PCO_2 are measured by the analyser, allowing calculation of $[HCO_3^-]$.

This approach assumes that PCO_2 and HCO_3^- are independent variables and becomes less robust when analysing complicated derangements, particularly metabolic acidosis. The Stewart approach, based on basic physico-chemical principles, while more complex, makes no such assumptions and has proven accurate and reliable in all circumstances.

Whatever the underlying cause(s) there are only 4 basic acid-base disturbances. These are respiratory acidosis and alkalosis and metabolic acidosis and alkalosis. Unfortunately life is not so simple and the actual picture may conceal an acute or chronic problem, a combination of two pathological processes or frequently a primary derangement partially or completely compensated for by the other system, e.g. a metabolic acidosis with respiratory compensation. Strictly speaking as this compensation is not a pathological process it should not be termed an alkalosis.

Using a systematic approach to the analysis the following questions should be addressed:

1. What is the pH? Is it outside the normal range?
   Is it low (acidaemia) or high (alkalaemia)?

The pH will, by definition, be within the normal range if the primary abnormality is fully compensated.

2. What is the serum bicarbonate, base excess and/or standard bicarbonate? Is a metabolic acidosis or alkalosis present?

3. What is the P_aco_2? Is there a respiratory component to the derangement?

The serum bicarbonate (normal 24) is derived from the H-H equation and is the actual concentration in the sample. As this is a variable of both the P_aco_2 and non-volatile acid production, various methods are described to attempt to clarify their relative contributions.

In 1960 Astrup described the concept of Standard Bicarbonate. This is the $[HCO_3^-]$ of the sample when in equilibrium with a gas mixture containing P_aco_2 5.3 kPa and P_ao_2 13.3 kPa at 37°C, thus eliminating abnormal respiration. The normal is around 24 mmol/l, less indicating metabolic acidosis and vice versa. The same concept can be applied to pH.

The standard bicarbonate is 17.1 mmol/l in the sample above, indicative of a significant metabolic acidosis.

Siggaard-Anderson and Engel, also in 1960, described the concept of Base Excess, again attempting to eliminate any respiratory component to the picture. Base excess is the concentration (mmol/l) of strong acid or base required to return a sample of whole blood (at 37°C and with $P_a co_2$ of 5.3 kPa) to a pH of 7.4. Originally this was calculated using nomograms derived from volunteer studies but this has been replaced by the Van Slyke equation, derived from theoretical concepts, but validated for in vitro calculations over a wide range of actual pCO_2. Base excess is a positive figure, indicating metabolic alkalosis while base deficit is negative and indicative of acidosis (normal -2 to $+2$).

Standard Base Excess is a further calculation attempting to convert the in vitro to an in vivo measurement and may be more representative.

A base deficit of 8.5 mmol/l (in the sample) is thus a second way of expressing the size of the metabolic acidosis. Discussion of base excess can be complicated by double negatives: a base deficit of 8.5 mmol/l is the same as a base excess of -8.5 mmol/l.

Respiratory disturbances

A primary respiratory disorder exists when the $P_a co_2$ is abnormal but not as compensation for another abnormality. In respiratory acidosis, pH is low while $P_a co_2$ is elevated, as is bicarbonate. Base excess and standard bicarbonate are within the normal range (by definition). Respiratory acidosis, when seen in acute respiratory failure indicates a serious, potentially life threatening condition.

Chronic CO_2 retainers – as seen in severe airways disease – in contrast often have a fully compensated blood gas picture. $P_a co_2$ is elevated but pH is normal. Renal compensation further elevates [HCO_3^-] and induces base excess and high standard bicarbonate.

Respiratory alkalosis is seen in conditions which induce hyperventilation. This can be acute (e.g. hypoxia or acute anxiety) or chronic (usually due to hypoxia). If uncompensated, pH is elevated and $P_a co_2$ is low, as is bicarbonate. Base excess and standard bicarbonate are normal.

The kidneys do not usually fully compensate for chronic respiratory alkalosis. Thus pH remains high or high normal, $P_a co_2$ remains low, as does bicarbonate. A moderate base deficit and slightly reduced standard bicarbonate complete the picture. Since only partial compensation is the norm, it is not difficult to conclude that the primary pathology is the respiratory alkalosis.

Metabolic disturbances

Metabolic alkalosis is a surprisingly common disturbance in the hospital population and is most commonly secondary to excessive gastrointestinal losses (vomiting) or due to diuretic therapy. Iatrogenic alkali administration is also important.

In acute metabolic alkalosis the pH, standard bicarbonate and base excess are all elevated. $P_a co_2$ will be in the normal range until significant respiratory compensation has occurred. As compensation involves hypoventilation, $P_a co_2$ will be elevated and bicarbonate rises further.

When considered logically a sustained metabolic alkalosis seems contradictory given the kidneys' ability to rapidly lose bicarbonate. Thus the condition will only be present if this ability is lost or inhibited. Acute renal failure will obviously inhibit compensation, particularly if the precipitating cause has resulted in significant volume depletion. More often the pathological process leading to the metabolic alkalosis will also induce significant electrolyte loss, particularly of chloride and potassium ions. Chloride ions are exchanged for bicarbonate ions in the kidney and this process is inhibited in hypochloraemic states. Thus typically these patients present with a hypochloraemic, hypokalaemic, metabolic alkalosis.

As many of the causes of metabolic alkalosis can be anticipated, prevention is frequently possible. This may involve the administration of H_2-antagonists to patients with high gastric losses, reducing diuretic therapy or providing adequate amounts of electrolyte replacements to patients at risk.

Management in the first instance, is adequate volume replacement and correction of electrolyte disturbances. This usually involves the administration of sodium chloride and potassium chloride solutions. Attention to the precipitating cause should proceed simultaneously.

Metabolic acidosis is a process leading to a fall in serum bicarbonate concentration. It is frequently seen in the critically ill and if unopposed, will lead to an acidaemia – a fall in pH below 7.36. The blood gas analysis also reveals a significant base deficit and low standard bicarbonate.

Some respiratory compensation is to be expected unless the patient is severely compromised. Hyperventilation lowers the $P_a co_2$ and with the consequent shift in equilibrium further lowers $[HCO_3^-]$.

The cause of acidosis may be clinically obvious (e.g. shock or renal failure) but cannot be reliably inferred from the blood gas analysis alone. For further insight into the underlying aetiology other indices must be examined. A helpful and widely used classification depends on the status of the anion gap.

Electrical neutrality in plasma is a fundamental principle and thus the total number of cations and anions must be equal. The major extracellular (measurable) cations are Na^+, K^+, Ca^{2+} and Mg^{2+} and anions are Cl^- and HCO_3^-. Unmeasured anions including albumin, phosphates, sulphates and other organic compounds normally total about 12 mmol/l, thus giving the anion gap. If a normal anion gap is present then HCO_3^- loss must have been replaced by Cl^-. If the anion gap has increased, then bicarbonate must have been replaced, at least in part, by another compound, usually an organic acid such as lactate.

There are a number of factors that may confound this simple approach in the critically ill. The patients frequently have a low serum albumin, which in itself reduces the anion gap and thus may mask the presence of an organic acid. Absolute values of the major serum electrolytes may also be low due to water overload.

Thus a slightly more thoughtful approach to the problem may be necessary and Stewart's (as discussed earlier), is most helpful.

Stewart found that three independent variables determine pH: $P_a co_2$, weak acid concentrations and strong (completely dissociated in solution) ion differences. $P_a co_2$ levels are more concerned with respiratory abnormalities. The most important strong ions are sodium and chloride and as the strong ion difference falls, so does pH: in other words Cl^- is an acidifying ion. This explains why normal saline is acidic and why excess administration of the same actually worsens a metabolic acidosis. A fall in albumin increases pH, also explained by Stewart's model.

A simplified application of the Stewart approach has been proposed that helps to eliminate some of the problems associated with the anion gap by looking at the chloride/sodium ratio. Thus, in a patient with a metabolic acidosis, a ratio <0.75 is highly predictive of the presence of abnormal tissue acids. Conversely a ratio >0.79 (a normal anion gap) suggests their absence. Between these variables a mixed picture is present – not uncommon in the intensive care unit.

What are the common causes of metabolic acidosis and how are they managed?

1. **Normal anion gap – high chloride/sodium ratio.** This is relatively uncommon but, in the acute setting, may be due to excessive HCO_3^- losses that occur, for instance, in the presence of gastro-intestinal fistula or diarrhoea. Excessive administration of normal saline solution, as discussed above, may be the primary cause. Other causes include a number of congenital or acquired metabolic disorders, including renal tubular acidosis. Specific management should be directed at the cause. If due to excess HCO_3^- loss, this can be replaced, if due to excess chloride administration, this can be withdrawn.

2. **Increased anion gap – low chloride/sodium ratio.** In these conditions abnormal acid or acids will be present. The most common precipitating conditions are:

   a. Lactic acidosis – Lactate is produced during the tissue metabolism of glucose in the presence of inadequate oxygen – anaerobic metabolism. Most commonly this is due to reduced tissue perfusion and is thus a feature of shock. In septic shock, lactic acidosis may be a function of abnormal cellular function and not just due to hypoxia.

   Most intensive care units now have the ability to measure lactate concentration within minutes, the normal being 0.6–1.8 mmol/l. Management includes attention to the underlying cause and active resuscitation of the patient with fluids and inotropes. The use of

16

alkalising agents is controversial. As lactate is largely eliminated within the liver, lactic acidosis may also occur with liver dysfunction. The lactate of 1.3 mmol/l in the sample above is of little significance.

b. Diabetic ketoacidosis – a degree of ketosis is normal in the fasting subject. Ketoacidosis occurs when a low insulin level results in excess, uninhibited production of ketones by the liver. These patients are also often severely dehydrated and may thus have an associated lactic acidosis. In the presence of shock, the main ketone produced is beta-hydroxybutyrate, which is not detected by conventional analytical techniques and thus ketosis can be missed. Management principally involves fluid and electrolyte administration, with insulin therapy to stop ketone production and reduce the blood glucose. Excessive administration of normal saline may replace one acidosis with another.

c. Renal failure – acidosis results from progressive accumulation of the acidic metabolic 'waste', normally excreted by this organ. The rate of progression depends on the severity of the renal failure and the catabolic state of the patient. Early intervention with renal replacement therapy may be life saving in the septic patient.

d. Salicylate poisoning – this causes a complex metabolic derangement with acidosis being due not only to the presence of salicylic acid, but also lactic acid, ketoacids and other organic compounds. Measurement of serum salicylate levels is usually diagnostic. Management includes basic resuscitation measures and volume expansion with normal saline. Glucose should also be given and any other electrolyte abnormality corrected. A forced alkaline diuresis using sodium bicarbonate is indicated in this condition.

e. Methanol and ethylene glycol poisoning – these compounds (both normally inert), become toxic when metabolised to organic acids. These intermediary metabolites may cause irreversible organ damage and death. Diagnosis relies on suspicion. Those poisoned may appear drunk, with a metabolic acidosis and increased serum osmolality, but with normal electrolytes (increased osmolar gap). Laboratory measurement of these alcohols is possible but treatment should not await this confirmation. These patients should be given ethanol (the preferred substrate for alcohol dehydrogenase), which will reduce toxic metabolite production. Early initiation of haemofiltration or dialysis may be life saving.

Finally, looking at our blood gas sample, the patient has both deranged gas exchange (severe acute lung injury) and a moderate metabolic acidosis (base deficit 8.5 mmol/l). The cause of the latter is unclear. Shock is unlikely with a normal lactate and ketosis unusual with minimally elevated blood glucose. Renal failure is possible but note the normal $[K^+]$.

Further reading

Durward A, et al. The value of the chloride:sodium ratio in differentiating the aetiology of metabolic acidosis. Intensive Care Med 2001; 27:828–835.

Matamis D and Papanikolaou G. Blood gas exchange. Int J Intensive Care. Winter 1998; 125–132.

Sirker AA, Rhodes A, Grounds RM and Bennett ED. Acid-base physiology: the 'traditional' and the 'modern' approaches. Anaesthesia 2002; 57:348–356.

Stewart PA. Modern quantitative acid-base chemistry. Can J Physiol Pharmacol 1983; 61:1444–1461.

16

17

Drugs used in anaesthesia and sedation

Mike Palmer

Anaesthetic agents

Volatile agents

These anaesthetic agents are highly volatile liquids which are allowed to vaporise in a stream of fresh gas (oxygen/air or oxygen/nitrous oxide) so that a given concentration by volume of the agent is ultimately inhaled. The concept of the minimum alveolar concentration (MAC) has been used to compare the potency of various agents. 1 MAC is the minimum alveolar concentration required to prevent movement of the patient in response to a standard surgical stimulus. The higher the potency of the agent the lower MAC will be. MAC values are additive and so a mixture of 2 volatile agents at concentrations of half MAC will produce the same result as 1 MAC for a single agent. MAC is however determined by other factors such as age and can be further reduced for all agents by using an opioid to provide analgesia. Volatile agents themselves appear to have no significant analgesic activity.

The volatile agents in use in the UK at present are *halothane* (in use since the 1960s), *enflurane*, *isoflurane*, *sevoflurane* and *desflurane*. *Halothane* and *sevoflurane* are sweet smelling and non-irritant and can be used to induce as well as maintain anaesthesia.

Effects on other systems

Hypotension	*Halothane* and *enflurane* produce myocardial depression and some vasodilatation. *Isoflurane* and *sevoflurane* produce hypotension mainly by vasodilatation. *Desflurane* also produces a fall in blood pressure but increasing concentration from 1 to 2 MAC results in a rise in blood pressure.
↑ Cerebral blood flow	This is a concern if intracranial pressure is elevated.
Arrhythmias	*Halothane* is associated with arrhythmias, particularly in the presence of high levels of circulating catecholamines.
Respiratory depression	All these agents depress respiration and also the response to hypercarbia and hypoxia.

Bronchodilatation
Relaxation of the gravid uterus

All these agents may precipitate malignant hyperpyrexia, a rare but potentially fatal elevation of body temperature.

The main route of excretion of these agents and thus recovery is via the lungs. However, up to 20% of *halothane* may be metabolised in the liver. *Halothane* has been linked to the development of hepatitis, particularly after multiple exposures, but the precise link is unclear.

Nitrous oxide/N₂O

A colourless, almost odourless gas. It is a poor anaesthetic agent alone as it has a MAC of >100% (as derived from experiments under 2 atmospheres pressure). It is therefore not possible to use N_2O as the sole anaesthetic agent as normally at least 30% oxygen is delivered during anaesthesia. It has analgesic properties and is used in a 50:50 mixture with oxygen as 'Entonox' for obstetric and emergency uses. Its use has been widespread as a 'carrier gas' for other anaesthetic agents, where it reduces the requirements of the volatile agents. However, its use has been associated with problems. It is a myocardial depressant, although this is unlikely to be a problem in people without cardiovascular disease. It diffuses into closed air spaces (in the gut, middle air and more dangerously a pneumothorax) faster than nitrogen diffuses out and so expands these spaces. If used for longer than a few hours it inhibits methionine synthase, which is involved in DNA synthesis and can lead to agranulocytosis. Furthermore, it is a greenhouse gas!

17

Intravenous anaesthetics

These drugs are used primarily to induce anaesthesia. They have a rapid onset of action (usually the time it takes to pass from the arm to the brain; the arm-brain circulation time) and after a single dose their effects are terminated by redistribution from the brain to other tissues. Some intravenous anaesthetics are also used for maintenance of anaesthesia and also sedation.

Sodium thiopentone is a barbiturate used in doses between 2 and 7 mg/kg and produces unconsciousness within 10–15 s, with consciousness returning after some 5–10 min due to redistribution. The actual elimination half life of thiopentone is 5–10 h and liver enzymes become saturated so repeated doses or intravenous infusions result in a very prolonged duration of action. It produces a period of apnoea and depression of respiration. It will also produce hypotension and this can be severe or even fatal in those patients who are hypovolaemic or have limited cardiac reserve. It has the advantage of being an anticonvulsant and also reduces intracranial pressure. It therefore has some use as an infusion in the management of intractable seizures or in patients with raised intracranial pressure (e.g. after head injury).

Propofol is di-isopropyl phenol and is presented in a white lipid emulsion, as it is insoluble in water. It is given in doses of 1.25–5 mg/kg. It can cause discomfort on injection but produces rapid loss of consciousness although muscle twitching and hiccuping can be seen in some patients. Its action is again terminated by redistribution but it has a short half-life and can be used as repeated boluses or an infusion for prolonged procedures, whilst allowing rapid full recovery. Its use is associated with apnoea, which may be of a longer duration than thiopentone and also hypotension, which may also be more marked than thiopentone and is due to vasodilatation. Airway reflexes are depressed to a greater extent than with thiopentone, allowing the insertion of a laryngeal mask airway without precipitating laryngospasm. Patients in whom anaesthesia is maintained with a propofol infusion appear to have a reduced incidence of postoperative nausea and vomiting.

Etomidate is administered in 0.2–0.3 mg/kg doses and has a rapid onset but often causes pain and discomfort on injection and a greater incidence of involuntary muscle movements than propofol. Its main advantage is that it produces less hypotension than either of the above agents and can be used for patients whose cardiovascular system is compromised. Recovery is rapid but can be associated with nausea and vomiting. Prolonged infusions of etomidate have been shown to cause adrenocortical suppression which may be fatal in the critically ill. This has not been shown to be significant after a single dose.

Ketamine has the advantage that it can be administered either intravenously or by intramuscular injection. Given intravenously in doses of 1–2 mg/kg it produces loss of consciousness within 1 min (slower than other agents) and after intramuscular injection of 5–10 mg/kg consciousness is lost in about 8–10 min. It has powerful amnesic and analgesic effects. Repeat doses or infusions can be used to maintain anaesthesia. It stimulates the sympathetic nervous system so that heart rate, cardiac output and blood pressure are maintained even in those patients who are hypovolaemic. There is also less respiratory depression than with the other agents. However, recovery can be associated with vivid dreams and hallucinations, although these can be minimised by using concurrent midazolam or other benzodiazepines. Its main uses are in children who have to undergo repeated, painful procedures and also in prehospital care to allow management of victims of road traffic accidents.

Midazolam is a benzodiazepine with a short half-life of 2 h. It is an anxiolytic and produces retrograde amnesia in patients. In higher doses it acts as a hypnotic. Low doses have little effect on the cardiovascular system but the higher doses can produce hypotension and respiratory depression. It is often given intravenously to provide sedation for procedures performed under local or regional anaesthesia and its use as a co-induction agent allows smaller doses of propofol to be used.

Neuromuscular blocking agents

Muscle relaxation and paralysis is used to facilitate intubation and allow surgical access which otherwise requires high concentrations of volatile agents. There are 2 classes of neuromuscular blocking agent, depolarising blockers and non-depolarising blockers.

Suxamethonium is the only depolarising blocker in use. Its structure is that of 2 acetylcholine (ACh) molecules joined via an ester link. It binds to ACh receptors at the neuromuscular junction resulting in muscle depolarisation (detected by muscle fasciculations clinically). However, suxamethonium is not metabolised by acetylcholinesterase so depolarisation persists and prevents further muscle activity. The effects wear off after about 5 min when suxamethonium diffuses away from the neuromuscular junction as it is cleared from the plasma by the action of the enzyme pseudocholinesterase. Patients with abnormal pseudocholinesterase activity may have a prolonged response lasting several hours.

Suxamethonium has a rapid onset and is mainly used in rapid sequence induction where intubation of the trachea is required rapidly after loss of consciousness (for example in patients with a full stomach). It can be associated with a number of adverse reactions such as profound bradycardia, dangerous elevations in plasma K^+ concentrations, histamine release, anaphylactoid reaction and malignant hyperpyrexia. It also produces muscular pains, particularly in young adults.

There are several drugs which bind competitively to the ACh receptor and produce non-fasciculating paralysis (non-depolarising blockers). They are all used to maintain muscle relaxation to allow abdominal surgery and in some patients to allow mechanical ventilation on intensive care. *Atracurium* and *vecuronium* are 2 drugs with a duration of action of about 20–30 min. Drugs with a longer duration of action (2 h) such as *pancuronium* are also used. *Atracurium* has the advantage in that it is metabolised by spontaneous Hoffman degradation in plasma and its elimination is not altered by hepatic or renal failure. *Rocuronium* is a relatively new agent which has a faster onset of action and can be used instead of suxamethonium to enable rapid endotracheal intubation, although at doses sufficient to allow intubation in around 30 seconds, it may take as long as 40 minutes to wear off.

Drugs and the autonomic nervous system

Many drugs which interact with the autonomic nervous system are used in anaesthesia. For example, *atropine* is used as a vagolytic agent to prevent bradycardia associated with various stimuli, such as intubation. (N.B. Although intubation often stimulates a stress response with associated tachycardia and hypertension, it is sometimes associated with excessive vagal stimulation due to the anatomic course of the vagus nerve. This can result in severe bradyarrhythmias in those with high vagal tone, e.g. children.) It is also used to dry up secretions that may affect the respiratory system. *Hyoscine* is used for similar reasons and is more sedative when given preoperatively. *Glycopyrrolate* is a quaternary ammonium molecule that has similar effects to atropine but does not cross the blood-brain barrier.

Neostigmine is an acetylcholinesterase inhibitor which is used to increase the concentration of acetylcholine available at the neuromuscular junction and so terminate the effects of competitive neuromuscular blocking drugs. It is administered with an anti-muscarinic such as atropine since profound bradycardia can result.

Various vasoactive drugs are also used. *Ephedrine* is used as an indirect sympathomimetic to increase release of noradrenaline from sympathetic neurons. It therefore increases heart rate and causes some vasoconstriction to reverse hypotension associated with anaesthesia. *Methoxamine* and *metaraminol* are direct α-agonists used for a similar purpose. They produce vasoconstriction without an increase in cardiac output and may actually

produce a bradycardia due to activation of baroreceptor reflexes.
(see Chapter 15: Inotropes for more detail)

Opioids

Morphine and other opioids are used extensively in anaesthesia. Morphine
remains the commonest drug for use in postoperative analgesia. *Fentanyl* is a
more potent opioid which can be used to obtund the hypertension and
tachycardia associated with intubation and surgical stimuli. As a single bolus
it has a duration of action of about 30 min but accumulates after prolonged
infusion. *Alfentanil* is similar although it has a shorter duration of action
(10 min) and may be used as an infusion with less risk of accumulation and
postoperative respiratory depression. *Remifentanil* is a more recent addition.
It has a very short duration of action even after prolonged infusions.

Sedation

Patients may require sedation for a number of reasons. For example during
invasive procedures, as premedication, before dental surgery and when
they are requiring ventilation in intensive care. Sedation involves
producing hypnosis without anaesthesia so the patient should maintain
verbal contact with the anaesthetist/operator at all times, although their
responses to command may be delayed. If sedated patients do not
respond, an overdose of the sedative agent has been given and the
patient is anaesthetised. It is often a beneficial side effect that the agents
used cause amnesia of an unpleasant procedure and this may persist after
the sedative effect has worn off.

   The practice of using more than one drug at a time has fallen into disuse
because of the danger of overdose from the combination used.
Benzodiazepines such as *midazolam* are most commonly used. It can be
given orally or intravenously, produces sedation and amnesia and is fairly
short acting. Intravenous increments of 1 mg of midazolam titrated to
clinical effect are often used, however it should be noted that some patients
(particularly the elderly) may become irritable and disorientated with only
modest doses. Overdose may be treated with the antagonist *flumazenil*.
Temazepam is used as a sedative at night although a newer benzodiazepine
receptor agonist *zopiclone* is being used increasingly frequently.
Benzodiazepines may cause respiratory and cardiovascular depression in the
elderly and can cause paradoxical excitation in both the elderly and children.

   Propofol can be used as sedation during surgery performed under local
or regional anaesthesia but care has to be taken that the patient does not
become anaesthetised. Propofol and midazolam, together with an opioid
for analgesia, are often used as sedatives on intensive care units to allow
patients to tolerate mechanical ventilation.

   Other drugs which have been used include *barbiturates* which have
largely been abandoned as they are dangerous in overdose and can have

prolonged duration of action. Anti-histamines such as *promethazine* and anti-cholinergics such as *hyoscine* have been used, particularly in premedication, but cause anti-muscarinic side effects. Anti-psychotic agents like *chlorpromazine* and *haloperidol* can be used to sedate the more disturbed patients but both have a number of adverse effects. *Ketamine* can be given to sedate patients for painful procedures as it has both analgesic and amnesic properties. It is good for changing burns dressings as it avoids the need for repeated anaesthetics.

> **Key points**
>
> 1. Volatile agents are used primarily to maintain anaesthesia but halothane and sevoflurane, which are not irritant can be used to induce anaesthesia.
>
> 2. Intravenous agents are used to induce anaesthesia, with propofol also being used to maintain anaesthesia as part of total intravenous anaesthetic techniques.
>
> 3. Neuromuscular blocking agents are used to facilitate endotracheal intubation and allow surgical access.
>
> 4. Opioids are used to obtund autonomic responses to surgical stimuli and airway manipulation as well as intra- and postoperative analgesia.
>
> 5. Drugs affecting the autonomic nervous system are used to prevent excess vagal stimulation and to correct hypotension produced by anaesthesia.
>
> 6. Sedative (hypnotic) drugs are given to patients for a number of reasons. Single agents should be used with minimal hangover and adverse effects. Amnesia may be a beneficial side effect. The patient should never completely lose consciousness.

17

Further reading

Calvey TN and Williams NE. Principles and Practice of Pharmacology for Anaesthetists, 3rd edn. Blackwell Science, 1997.

Sasada M and Smith S. Drugs in Anaesthesia & Intensive Care, 2nd edn. Oxford University Press, 1997.

18

Local anaesthetics

Sue Abdy

For thousands of years native South American Indians chewed the leaves of Coca plants to produce mild euphoria, stimulation and alertness. The numbing effect of chewing these leaves on the mouth and tongue was known long before cocaine was isolated. It was first used clinically by Carl Köller, an ophthalmologist from Vienna in 1884. He demonstrated that dropping cocaine into the eye could produce reversible corneal anaesthesia. However, it was not until 1904 when procaine was synthesised, that significant advances in local anaesthetic techniques could be made. This is due to cocaine being unsuitable for anything other than topical use, due to its systemic toxicity, central nervous system stimulation, addictive properties and tendency to cause allergic reactions.

Pharmacology

1. Structure

All local anaesthetic agents have a tertiary amine group linked to an aromatic group. They are classified as either esters or amides depending on the linkage between them.

Examples of esters:
  Cocaine
  Procaine
  Amethocaine
  Benzocaine
Examples of amides:
  Prilocaine
  Lignocaine
  Bupivacaine
  Ropivacaine

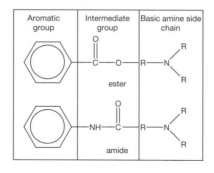

Esters are broken down by plasma cholinesterases and are more allergenic, but cause less toxicity. Amides are metabolised by the liver and cause fewer allergic reactions, but have greater systemic toxicity.

2. Mechanism of action

Local anaesthetic agents work by reversibly blocking the fast sodium channels in the cell membrane of neurons, thereby preventing propagation of action potentials and thus preventing nerve transmission. The sodium channels are blocked from inside the nerve. The local anaesthetic has to get through the cell membrane to work and as a result must be lipid soluble i.e. in its non-ionised state. However, to block the ion channel local anaesthetics need to be in the ionised form (water soluble). Hence, they need to be able to change their ionic state once inside the cell. Local anaesthetics are weak bases (i.e. they attract protons or hydrogen ions). They can thus exist in two states; either the acid (ionised) state or the basic (non-ionised) state.

18

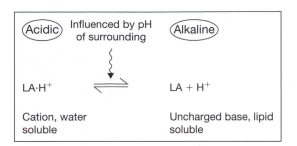

These two forms are always in equilibrium but the ratio of each depends on the pKa (dissociatic constant) of the local anaesthetic agent and the pH of its surroundings.

The pKa of a substance is the pH at which the ratio of ionised to non-ionised molecules is 1:1 (i.e. the drug is 50% ionised).

$$pKa = pH, \text{ when } [base] = [acid] \text{ or } [LA] = [LA \cdot H^+]$$

Small changes in pH lead to large changes in the proportion of drug that is ionised. To be useful clinically (i.e. in a form that is injectable), local anaesthetics need to be water soluble and are presented in an acid solution as the hydrochloride salt. The pKa of lignocaine (lidocaine) is 7.7 and the acid solution has a pH of 6. Using the Henderson-Hasselbalch equation:

$$pH = pKa + \frac{LA \text{ (base)}}{LA \cdot H^+ \text{ (acid)}}$$

This means that in a syringe containing lignocaine hydrochloride, 99% of the total is in the ionised form and only 1% is in the non-ionised form. This maintains water solubility. Once injected into the tissues, where the pH is 7.4, the proportion of drug that remains ionised drops to 76% of the total. Therefore 24% is in the non-ionised (lipid soluble) form and is thus able to diffuse passively down the concentration gradient across the nerve cell membrane. Once inside the cell the pH drops to 7.1, which pushes the equilibrium between ionised and non-ionised drug back towards the ionised form (86% of the total). This has two effects. Firstly, it means the vast majority of drug inside the cell is in the active form, able to pass into and block the sodium channels. Secondly, it reduces the amount of non-ionised drug inside the cell thereby increasing the concentration gradient across the cell membrane thus allowing more to diffuse inside.

A. Speed of onset
Depends on the following:

- site and type of the nerve
- proximity of the injection

18

■ pKa of the local anaesthetic agent

■ acidity of the surroundings

A nerve may be blocked at any level from the spinal cord within the dura to the sensory receptors at the periphery. The local anaesthetic must diffuse into the cell to produce its effect. The speed with which this occurs will depend on the degree of myelination of the nerve, the size of the nerve and the relative position of the fibre within the nerve. Small, unmyelinated sympathetic nerves are blocked more easily than medium sized pain, temperature and touch fibres, which in turn are more susceptible than large, myelinated pressure, proprioception and motor fibres. As explained above, the speed at which local anaesthetic agents can diffuse into the cell is highly dependent on the agent's pKa. The lower the pKa the more non-ionised form is available to diffuse into the cell. If the pH of the tissues is lower than normal, for example when infection is present, then less of the agent is in the non-ionised form and the onset is much slower (in highly acidic, infected tissues, the local anaesthetic may not work at all). Likewise, if the agent is injected with alkali then more is available and onset will be more rapid.

B. Potency
The more lipid-soluble a local anaesthetic agent is the more potent it becomes.

C. Duration of action
Related to the following factors:

■ dose

■ local blood flow

■ intrinsic vasoactivity

■ vasoactive additives

■ protein binding

■ local drug metabolism

Obviously, the more drug that is injected the longer the duration is likely to be: total dose = volume × concentration. However, duration is also dependent on how long the drug remains in the tissues. Ester local anaesthetics for example, are rapidly metabolised by plasma cholinesterases and tend to have a shorter duration of action than amides, which are metabolised in the liver. How quickly the drug is removed depends on the vascularity of the tissues, which is altered by the intrinsic vasoactivity of the agent and also the vasoactivity of any additives, such as adrenaline (epinephrine). Local infection causes vasodilatation resulting in faster removal under these conditions. Protein binding also affects removal as protein bound drug cannot be metabolised.

18

Physicochemical and pharmacokinetic properties of local anaesthetic agents

	Lipid solubility	Relative potency	Protein binding (%)	Duration of action	pKa	Onset
Esters						
Amethocaine	High	4	75	Long	8.5	Slow
Procaine	Low	0.5	6	Short	8.9	Slow
Amides						
Bupivacaine	High	4	96	Long	8.1	Slow
Lignocaine	Medium	1	64	Medium	7.7	Rapid
Prilocaine	Medium	1	55	Medium	7.9	Rapid
Ropivacaine	Medium	3	95	Long	8.1	Medium

Complications of local anaesthetics

18

A. Systemic toxicity

This is mainly due to the membrane stabilising effects on other cells, especially the heart and central nervous system.

Increasing serum concentration of local anaesthetic	CNS symptoms	CVS symptoms
	Tingling around the mouth and tongue	
	Tinnitus, visual disturbance	
	Light-headedness	
	Tremor and agitation	
	Slurred speech	
	Muscle twitching	Myocardial depression
	Loss of consciousness, coma	Resistant cardiac arrhythmias
	Respiratory arrest	Ventricular arrest

Systemic toxicity results from either accidental intravenous injection or systemic absorption of a toxic amount.

Treatment of systemic toxicity:

1. Stop injection

2. ABC principles of resuscitation

3. Treat convulsions if persistent

4. Treat cardiac dysrhythmias if cardiac output is compromised

5. Correct any ensuing electrolyte abnormalities

B. Allergic reactions

These are more commonly associated with esters. Esters can also cause cross-sensitivity (i.e. if a patient is allergic to one ester they are likely to react to the others). Amides themselves rarely cause allergic reactions. When they do, they do not tend to cause cross-sensitivity and it is usually safe to use other amides in such patients. However, the preservatives used in multi-dose vials of amide local anaesthetic agents (such as methyl hydroxybenzoate) have a relatively high incidence of causing allergic reactions. It is therefore safer to use solutions without preservatives.

C. Local infection

As with any invasive procedure, introduction or spread of infection during injection of local anaesthetic is always a potential complication. This can be minimised by meticulous aseptic technique and sterile equipment.

D. Trauma

Damage to nerves due to:

- Direct needle puncture

- Intra-neural injection

- Nerve compression due to poor positioning of patient

- Inadvertent thermal injury to anaesthetised area

- Damage to blood vessels causing haematomata

- Needle breakage

- Ischaemia and necrosis after incorrect use of a vasoconstrictor around an end artery, or due to the pressure effect of injected local anaesthetic

E. Unintentional blockade of other nerves

For example: Horner's syndrome after interscalene block (may be inevitable)
Femoral nerve block after ilioinguinal block
Phrenic nerve block can also occur during brachial plexus block

F. Methaemoglobinaemia

Prilocaine is metabolised to *o*-toluidine. This causes oxidation of haemoglobin which is then less able to bind oxygen. Methaemoglobin is

18

dark; this causes patients to appear cyanosed and causes inaccurate readings with pulse oximetry. Patients become symptomatic, complaining of dyspnoea and headache if levels reach 20%, particularly if the rate of formation is rapid. Methaemoglobinaemia is rare unless more than 600 mg of prilocaine is administered. Fetal haemoglobin is more sensitive and prilocaine is therefore not used in obstetric anaesthesia.

Commonly used local anaesthetic agents

Lignocaine (Lidocaine)
- Amide local anaesthetic agent and class Ib anti-arrhythmic drug.

- Rapid onset and medium duration of action.

- Maximum safe dose   3 mg/kg (plain)

    7 mg/kg (with adrenaline).

- Uses:

  - Local infiltration.

  - Topical anaesthesia of mucous membranes (e.g. the mouth, pharynx, larynx, respiratory tract and urethra).

  - Epidural anaesthesia (tolerance and reduced effect occurs with prolonged infusion).

  - Topical anaesthesia of the skin (in EMLA® cream).

Bupivacaine
- Amide local anaesthetic agent.

- Slow onset with a prolonged duration of action.

- Maximum safe dose 2 mg/kg.

- Particularly cardiotoxic (since it enters the Na^+ channel *fast*, but diffuses out *slowly*.

- Now available as a single enantiomer 'levobupivacaine' (Chirocaine®), claimed to have a much safer side effect profile.

- Uses:

  - Spinal and epidural anaesthesia.

  - Nerve and plexus blockade.

  - Local infiltration.

Other agents include prilocaine, ropivacaine, cocaine and tetracaine (amethocaine).

Two topical local anaesthetic creams often used on the wards are EMLA® and Ametop®.

18

EMLA® cream

■ Eutectic Mixture of Local Anaesthetics. (Eutectic means that the melting point of each agent is lowered by the presence of the other.)

■ 2.5% prilocaine and 2.5% lignocaine (non-ionised state).

■ Applied to unbroken skin and covered with an occlusive dressing.

■ Provides topical analgesia for venepuncture and cannulation after about 60 min. Effect declines after removal.

AMETOP®

■ 4% Tetracaine (amethocaine) gel.

■ Applied to unbroken skin and covered with an occlusive dressing.

■ Provides topical anaesthesia for phlebotomy and cannulation after 30–45 min, lasting 4–6 h.

18

Key points

1. Local anaesthetics are both lipid soluble (to cross membranes) and water soluble (to diffuse to the Na^+ channel).

2. The degree of ionisation depends on the pH of the surroundings and the pKa of the individual local anaesthetic.

3. Amide local anaesthetics are generally very safe, however remember the maximal safe doses and central nervous system and cardiovascular system manifestations of systemic toxicity.

Further reading

Local anaesthetic agents. In: Calvey TN, Williams NE. Principles and Practice of Pharmacology for Anaesthetists. Blackwell Science, Oxford 1997, pp 284–316.

19

Monitoring used in the perioperative period

Ian Bridgland and Katrina Williams

Introduction

The perioperative period carries increased risk of patient morbidity and mortality. This risk can arise from the patient's preexisting medical problems, the pathophysiology of the surgical illness, from surgical or investigative procedures and from anaesthetic interventions. Perioperative monitoring has evolved as one strategy to minimise this risk. The scope of monitoring has dramatically increased in recent years to the point where there appears to be a bewildering array of monitoring possibilities available. An adequate understanding of the available monitoring tools is necessary to allow the clinician to obtain the information necessary to guide treatment, whilst at the same time minimising the risk of harm to the patient. This chapter describes some of the more commonly employed types of monitoring and outlines their uses and limitations. Patients are monitored by clinical observation supplemented by the use of selected monitoring devices.

Clinical observation

The importance of clinical observation cannot be overemphasised. A wide variety of information is available to the perceptive clinician, although one should be wary of interpreting clinical signs in isolation. The environment in which a patient is assessed, whether it be the emergency room, an inpatient ward or the operating theatre may provide additional challenges making accurate clinical observation difficult. Some of the types of information that may be obtained are listed below:

Oxygenation status
Cyanosis may be evident by a change in skin or blood colour. It is a sign of hypoxaemia and is an emergency. Cyanosis is only visible when 5 g/dl of deoxygenated haemoglobin is circulating, so might not be seen at all when anaemia and hypoxia coexist.

Cardiovascular system
Poor peripheral perfusion is suggested by a cold, pale periphery with delayed capillary refill. Pallor of the skin or conjunctiva may also indicate anaemia. Auscultation of the heart sounds provides more information about heart rate and rhythm as well as many cardiac disorders.

Respiratory function and airway patency
The simplest checks of ventilation are the breathing rate and the observation of adequate bilateral chest expansion. This can be confirmed by auscultation of the lungs. Auscultation of the lungs also assists in the diagnosis of pneumothorax, pulmonary oedema and secretions and aids in the detection of misplaced endotracheal tubes (e.g. inadvertent intubation of a bronchus).

Renal function

Satisfactory urine output reflects adequate renal perfusion and function. The perioperative use of diuretics should of course be taken into account.

Basic monitoring devices

Modern monitoring devices co-ordinate the measurement and display of several physiological parameters within a single instrument. Present best monitoring practice is to measure several parameters and interpret them in combination with clinical observation. Caution is required when interpreting any measured physiological parameter in isolation, as there are situations when each of them may be unreliable. A number of potential problems exist with the use of any piece of electrical monitoring equipment. Power failure or accidental electrical disconnection may result in loss of monitoring function. Furthermore, internal equipment failure may occur which is generally beyond the ability of the user to repair. Problems in interfacing the monitoring equipment to the patient may arise, such as cable or probe disconnection, cable damage and cable tangling. Interfacing problems are particularly likely to occur when transferring or repositioning a patient. Finally, faulty electrical equipment may represent a hazard to both patient and staff.

Pulse oximetry

Description

Pulse oximetry measures the percentage of haemoglobin combined with oxygen in the arterial circulation. The amount of light of any given wavelength absorbed by haemoglobin varies, depending on whether or not the haemoglobin is combined with oxygen. Pulse oximeters employ two different light wavelengths (660 nm in the visible spectrum and 940 nm in the infrared range) to allow a calculation of the proportion of oxygenated haemoglobin. The display of this measurement usually comprises a waveform, a numerical estimate of arterial oxygen saturation and the pulse rate. An audible tone timed to the pulse rate is usually available together with threshold alarms for low saturation and high and low pulse rates.

Indications

Pulse oximetry is used to ensure adequate arterial oxygenation, and is more sensitive than clinical observation for detecting hypoxia. It is used routinely during the induction and maintenance of anaesthesia (whether general anaesthesia, local anaesthesia or sedative technique) and in the recovery room. Other routine applications are in intensive care and during transport of the critically ill. The single probe connection to the patient makes pulse oximetry easy to set up.

19

Disadvantages

The trend towards hypoxia may be well advanced before it is detected as a significant fall in oxygen saturation. This is because the oxyhaemoglobin curve is relatively flat for arterial oxygen tensions above 10 kPa. There are a number of situations where inaccurate measurements of oxygen saturation may arise:

i. A poor pulsatile signal may arise from factors such as coloured nail varnish and reduced peripheral perfusion.

ii. Interference to the signal may be caused by strong light, diathermy or motion.

iii. Other types of haemoglobin and circulating pigments may cause abnormal readings. Carboxyhaemoglobin produces a measurement tending towards 90% saturation, whilst methaemoglobin tends towards 85%.

iv. Measurements outside the calibration range of the equipment (usually less than 50% saturation) may be inaccurate.

Non-invasive blood pressure monitoring

Description

The term 'non-invasive blood pressure' or NIBP generally refers to the use of an automated oscillotonometric method to measure blood pressure via a pneumatic limb cuff. The cuff usually encircles the upper arm, although the lower limb is also suitable. This technique involves inflating the pneumatic cuff to above systolic blood pressure and then slowly deflating it to atmospheric pressure. As the cuff pressure decreases, pressure oscillations of increasing magnitude will be noted within the cuff. The measurement process is automated and a variety of measurement time intervals is usually offered, together with threshold alarms for high and low systolic and diastolic pressures. It is important to select the correct cuff size in order to obtain accurate measurements.

Indications

Non-invasive blood pressure measurement has become enormously popular because the operator is free to carry out other activities whilst regular measurements are taken. Understandably, non-invasive blood pressure measurement has become the standard for perioperative blood pressure measurement.

Disadvantages

Two categories of problem may arise from non-invasive blood pressure measurement. These are patient injury and measurement inaccuracy. Injury to the limb caused by the repetitive inflation of

19

the cuff may manifest as neurological injury (particularly the ulnar nerve) or petechial skin haemorrhages under the cuff. Patients frequently complain of discomfort associated with high cuff pressures. Measurement errors occur in a wide variety of circumstances, such as shivering, gross limb movements, incorrect cuff size, arrhythmias and peripheral vascular disease.

Electrocardiography

Description
The normal sequence of atrial and ventricular contraction gives rise to characteristic electrical potentials measurable on the body surface. This electrical activity can be detected by electrodes placed on the skin and processed for display and analysis. There are a number of different ways of capturing and processing these signals:

i. Intermittent detailed snapshots of electrical activity are provided by the familiar 12-lead electrocardiogram (ECG). There are usually ten electrical connections made to the patient and electrical activity is sampled over a brief period.

ii. The term ECG monitoring refers to the continuous real-time capture of ECG information. This is usually made available as one or more waveforms on a display unit. Rapid changes in heart rate and rhythm can be identified, and acute changes in waveform morphology associated with ischaemia can be detected. The commonest monitoring systems involve three or five patient electrodes. Modern instruments employ alarm systems to alert the operator to high and low heart rates as well as dangerous arrhythmias.

iii. Holter monitoring and exercise electrocardiography are two further applications. During Holter monitoring, ECG signals over a 24 or 48 h period are stored for retrospective analysis. During exercise electrocardiography, a continuous 12-lead recording is usually made and is used to guide the progress of the investigation and is analysed retrospectively.

Indications
The ECG has become established as an important preoperative screening tool. Printouts of 12-lead ECGs are often used in conjunction with history and clinical examination to guide further cardiovascular investigation. The screening value of the ECG lies in its ability to detect arrhythmias, conduction defects and signs of past and present ischaemia. Holter monitoring and exercise electrocardiography may be useful in preoperative investigations where there is evidence or suspicion of cardiac disease. Requests for these investigations are usually best made in consultation with a cardiologist.

19

Disadvantages

There are a number of problems associated with ECG monitoring which emphasise the fact that abnormal results should never be interpreted in isolation:

i. The presence of a normal ECG signal provides no information about cardiac output. It is possible to have no cardiac output and a satisfactory ECG signal, for example in pulseless electrical activity (PEA, previously known as electromechanical dissociation, EMD).

ii. Multiple patient connections increase the risk of incorrect electrode connections, which may be misinterpreted. The chance of accidental lead disconnection is also increased.

iii. It may be difficult to obtain satisfactory adhesion or electrical contact of the electrodes to moist or oily skin.

iv. Measurement artefacts can arise from a variety of sources including muscle activity (particularly shivering), faults in the electrodes or leads or any source of electrical fields in the environment. Considerable design effort has gone into reducing measurement artefacts.

Temperature measurement

Description

The highly perfused tissues of the body including the brain, heart, liver and kidneys constitute the core thermal compartment. The temperature of this compartment is usually stable and slightly higher than the rest of the body at 36.5–37.5°C. Body temperature can be measured at a number of different sites and there are several different measurement technologies available. An important factor when choosing a measurement site is how well it correlates to core body temperature. Some commonly used sites together with their advantages and disadvantages are listed below:

i. Axilla – This site is convenient and carries a low risk of complications, however there may be poor correlation to core temperature. Furthermore, the axilla may take up to 15 min to reflect changes in core temperature. It is particularly useful in children who may not tolerate the use of other sites. The site lends itself to continuous and intermittent measurement techniques.

ii. Oral cavity – This requires a co-operative patient and is suited to intermittent use. The probe should be placed under the tongue on either side of the frenulum and the mouth closed until the temperature has stabilised. The measurement may be affected by recent consumption of hot or cold food or drinks.

iii. Rectum – The rectum may be difficult to access, particularly in trauma cases or intra-operatively. This site is usually the least acceptable to

19

patients and staff. The correlation to core temperature is less accurate when compared to the nasopharyngeal or oesophageal sites, and may be falsely elevated by gut bacterial activity.

iv. Tympanic membrane – The commonest method for measuring temperature at the tympanic membrane utilises infrared thermometry and the following points relate only to this technique. This site provides good correlation and rapid equilibration with core temperature. Arguably, this technique should only be used in alert patients to minimise the risk of insertion trauma. Gentle posterior traction on the ear straightens the external canal improving measurement accuracy. User related measurement errors relate to inadequate insertion of the probe, however the presence of earwax should not affect the measurement. Currently available infrared tympanic membrane temperature monitors provide intermittent measurements.

v. Nasopharynx and oesophagus – These measurement routes are applicable to intubated and sedated patients and are potentially the best sites for continuous temperature measurement.

vi. Skin – The temperature of the skin is highly variable and is affected by ambient temperature and local blood flow. As such it is an unreliable site for measuring core temperature. However, there are situations where skin temperature is deliberately measured to provide an indication of the adequacy of peripheral perfusion. This is particularly useful in children.

Indications

19

Several important conditions can give rise to changes in body temperature outside of the normal range in the perioperative period. Causes of hyperthermia include sepsis, adverse reactions to drugs and blood products and less commonly hyperthyroidism and malignant hyperthermia. Similarly, there are conditions that cause or contribute to hypothermia. These include cold intravenous fluid or blood therapy, environmental exposure and any factor that impairs an individual's normal physiological temperature regulatory mechanisms such as anaesthesia or reduced level of consciousness from any other cause. Temperature measurement is therefore important both for detecting abnormal changes in body temperature as well as guiding interventions aimed at restoring normal temperature. For these reasons temperature monitoring has become routine in the perioperative period.

Capnometry

Description

Capnometry involves the continuous breath-by-breath measurement of carbon dioxide concentration at a point close to the patient's mouth. It is a more specialised form of monitoring and is usually only found in the operating theatre and critical care areas. Capnometry is usually only practical when a patient is intubated because of the need to accurately sample their respiratory gas. Measured concentration of carbon dioxide is usually plotted against time on a graphical display – hence the more commonly used term capnography. The minimum and maximum amplitudes of the resulting waveform generally corresponds to the inspired and end tidal carbon dioxide concentrations. As with most other measured physiological parameters, threshold alarms are available to draw attention to high and low end tidal carbon dioxide as well as high values of inspired carbon dioxide.

Invasive pressure monitoring

General principles

There are many clinical situations where it is desirable to directly measure a pressure within the body. An example of this would be a dehydrated patient with bowel obstruction where measurement of central venous pressure helps to guide preoperative fluid resuscitation. Less common examples include intracranial pressure monitoring in head injury and pulmonary artery catheterisation in very severe cardiovascular disease. When a patient is sufficiently unstable to require invasive pressure monitoring, they are usually admitted to a high dependency or intensive care ward. In this way such patients are managed by staff who are not only accustomed to the specialised equipment required, but also to the care of patients with acute severe illness. There are two methods of invasive pressure measurement: simple manometric techniques and more complex electronic methods.

A manometer is a device which represents pressure by the height of a column of fluid above a reference point. As the measured pressure increases, the fluid is forced higher in the column against gravity. A graduated scale on the column allows the operator to read off the pressure directly from the height of the fluid meniscus. At the minimum it consists of a fluid filled catheter, which makes direct connection to the blood vessel or tissue being measured and also to the base of a graduated fluid column. The base of the column is set to the same height as the reference point of interest, for example the mid-axillary line (as an estimate of right atrial pressure). A manometer is a simple and inexpensive piece of equipment, but requires care in its use to avoid errors. It lends itself to intermittent measurement of slowly changing pressures within the range 0–100 cmH$_2$O such as central venous pressure. It is not suitable for larger pressures such as those found in the arterial circulation and does not allow automated recording or alarm generation.

Whilst electronic methods of invasive pressure monitoring involve complex equipment, the overall principles are relatively simple and are outlined in the diagram in the next page.

19

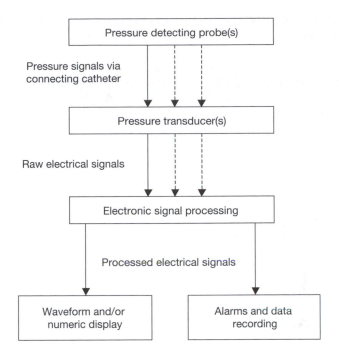

The example of central venous pressure is considered again to explain the various components of an electronic pressure monitoring system. In this case the pressure-detecting probe is the central venous line. The pressure in the central vein in which the line is placed is transmitted along the lumen of the line and through a fluid filled catheter connected to a pressure transducer. Here the changes in pressure transmitted via the fluid are converted to an electrical signal, which travels on to the signal-processing unit. This raw electrical signal is then modified into a form suitable for visual display. This may be a pressure vs time waveform, a numeric display of the mean pressure or both. The capability to measure pressure in this way is usually incorporated into a multi-function monitor that can simultaneously carry out other functions such as pulse oximetry and electrocardiography. Usually, such a monitor can measure and display several pressure sources at once and threshold alarms limits can be set to alert the practitioner to abnormal values.

Another important component of any electronic invasive pressure monitoring system is a means to continually flush the pressure conduit and probe to prevent damping or obstruction due to blood clot. This is usually achieved by having a bag of heparinised saline pressurised to 300 mmHg connected to the transducer end of the conduit via a narrow constriction. The calibre of the constriction is designed so that 2–4 mL/h of saline flushes the system without influencing the pressure measurement. A means to rapidly flush the system is usually also provided.

Invasive arterial pressure monitoring

Description

The pressure-detecting probe for arterial monitoring is a cannula placed percutaneously into an artery. The radial artery is usually selected because of convenience and a low incidence of complications. The technique of arterial cannulation is similar to venous cannulation and is ideally learned from an experienced clinician. The diameter of cannula used peripherally is usually limited to 20 gauge in the adult.

The information obtained from invasive arterial blood pressure (IABP) monitoring is frequently displayed as a pressure vs time waveform as well as numerical values of systolic, mean and diastolic arterial pressure.

Indications

The need for IABP monitoring arises in two broad groups of patients:

i. The patient's condition may predispose to large, sudden changes in blood pressure in the perioperative period that are important to detect rapidly. Examples of such conditions include major trauma and severe preexisting cardiovascular disease.

ii. The planned surgery may possibly precipitate major haemodynamic instability in a previously stable patient. This can be due to several causes including blood loss, large fluid shifts, or surgical manipulation of important components of the cardiovascular system such as the heart or major blood vessels.

iii. Patients undergoing cardiopulmonary bypass. These patients do not have pulsative blood flow. Traditional methods of recording blood pressure rely on oscillation and pulsation. The only way of assessing whether cardiopulmonary bypass is providing adequate perfusion pressure is by means of invasive arterial pressure monitoring.

In the patient groups listed above, rapid detection of blood pressure changes is important to guide management. Therapeutic interventions may include vasoactive and inotropic drugs with durations of action of only a few minutes. This clearly necessitates continuous blood pressure measurement to allow accurate titration. Another advantage of IABP monitoring in these patient groups is that they may have blood pressures below the measurement range of NIBP systems.

Another indication for IABP monitoring is the requirement to repeatedly sample arterial blood. Arterial blood can also be used where a venous sample would otherwise be required, such as for haematological or biochemical analysis.

19

Central venous pressure monitoring

Description

Central venous pressure (CVP) monitoring requires an intravenous catheter sited with its tip in the superior or inferior vena cava. Insertion sites include the internal jugular, subclavian and femoral veins as well as the veins of the cubital fossa in the upper limb. Central vein cannulation requires a degree of technical skill and an awareness of the possible complications. The various insertion techniques are not covered here and (as with arterial cannulation) these are best learned from an experienced practitioner. A number of different central venous catheters will be seen in clinical practice, varying in length, diameter and number of lumens. The information obtained from CVP monitoring is usually displayed as a pressure vs time waveform as well as a numerical value of mean CVP.

Indications

Central venous catheters are commonly inserted with the aim of measuring central venous pressure. This measurement is used to guide fluid therapy, particularly when other indicators of intravascular volume such as blood pressure and urine output are difficult to interpret. This is a common situation in critically ill patients. CVP measurement may also be used in patients with preexisting disease who would be poorly tolerant of significant changes in blood volume perioperatively. Examples of such diseases include cardiac and renal impairment.

In addition to CVP measurement, there are a number of other indications for inserting a central venous catheter. These are listed below:

i. Where peripheral intravenous access is difficult or impossible

ii. Where prolonged access is required for intravenous drug therapy

iii. When an administered drug is highly irritant to a peripheral vein, e.g. vancomycin, potassium.

iv. For repeated venous blood sampling

Problems

There are some important groups of problems associated with CVP monitoring and these are outlined below:

i. Complications of catheter insertion: These include local tissue trauma and haematoma, pneumothorax (especially for subclavian vein insertion), inadvertent arterial cannulation, air embolism and cardiac arrhythmias. The catheter tip may also fail to enter the caval veins and travel peripherally resulting in erroneous CVP measurements.

ii. Problems related to duration of use: The longer a central venous catheter remains *in situ*, the greater the risk of line associated sepsis

19

163

and thrombus formation. Furthermore a catheter tip lying in the right heart may over time erode the heart wall.

iii. Problems caused by line access: Because CVP may be below atmospheric pressure in some circumstances, accessing the line introduces the risk of air embolism. There is also a risk of introducing micro-organisms into the catheter each time it is accessed. Careful access technique is required to avoid these complications.

The pulmonary artery catheter

Description

Pulmonary artery (PA) catheterisation involves the percutaneous placement of a balloon-tipped catheter, the tip of which is introduced into a branch of the pulmonary artery via the right heart.

Indications

The use of a PA catheter is clearly a highly specialised type of monitoring and its use is limited to critical care areas and the operating room. It provides information about cardiac output, systemic and pulmonary vascular resistance, pulmonary artery pressures and pulmonary capillary occlusion pressure. Widely differing opinions as to the usefulness of PA catheters are likely to be encountered amongst practitioners, with some feeling that the associated risks rarely outweigh the benefits. A detailed description of PA catheters is outside the scope of this chapter.

Further reading

1 Recommendations for Standards of Monitoring during Anaesthesia and Recovery. Association of Anaesthetists, London, 2000. www.aagbi.org

2 Al-Shaik B, Stacey S. Essentials of Anaesthetic Equipment. Churchill Livingstone, London, 2001.

20

Deep vein thrombosis and thrombo-embolic disease prophylaxis

Jonathan Hudsmith

Background

Deep vein thrombosis (DVT) is difficult to diagnose clinically and its frequency has therefore been underestimated. Less than 20% of patients with proven pulmonary embolism (PE) have clinical features compatible with venous thrombosis in the legs.

Clinical features/symptoms of DVT are:

- Asymptomatic, presenting with clinical features of pulmonary embolism.

- Pain, swelling and redness in the calf, often associated with engorged superficial veins. The affected side may also be warmer and ankle oedema may be a feature.

Homan's sign of pain in the calf on dorsiflexion of the foot is often present. This is not diagnostic and occurs with many diseases affecting the calf. Testing for Homan's sign is not recommended as it may displace a thrombosis already present.

Thromboembolism in lower limb venous systems usually occurs as a complication of major surgery or of a serious illness.

Without anti-thrombotic prophylaxis, objective diagnostic measures have shown that 8–15% of patients develop venous thrombosis after major general surgery, 36–60% after surgery for hip fracture, 47–57% after total hip replacement and 40–80% after total knee replacement.

The frequency of DVT is less well documented in medical patients. A study using colour Doppler imaging detected an unexpectedly high rate of DVT of 33% in patients in an intensive care unit (48% of these cases were proximal leg thromboses). In addition, DVT occurs in 50% of patients following a cerebral vascular accident, and in one third of patients with a myocardial infarction.

Thrombosis of deep leg veins is serious since proximal vein thrombosis is the cause of fatal pulmonary embolism implicated in about 2 in 1,000 postoperative deaths each year. Most patients who die from PE do so within 30 min of the acute event, often too soon to make a correct diagnosis, or start treatment.

PE can occur with any deep vein thrombosis, but is most common with an iliofemoral thrombosis and occurs rarely with thromboses confined to the veins below the knee. Spread thrombosis proximally can occur without the development of symptoms or clinical signs. It is therefore essential to carefully establish the extent of the thrombosis.

The only effective treatment is prevention and prophylaxis should be offered to all patients at risk.

Diagnosis

Three tests have good accuracy for diagnosing DVT in *symptomatic* patients – venography, impedance plethysmography and duplex venous ultrasound (B-mode imaging). In most patients with clinically suspected DVT, venous

20

ultrasound is the diagnostic method of choice. In addition, the D-dimer blood test has high sensitivity and moderate specificity as a diagnostic test for venous thrombosis. The D-dimer test is often false positive after surgery or trauma, thereby limiting its diagnostic value in perioperative medicine.

Computed tomography and magnetic resonance imaging are useful diagnostic tools and are most sensitive for the suspected thrombosis of pelvic veins. Venography, although invasive, is the 'gold standard' diagnostic procedure. Duplex ultrasound is the best non-invasive diagnostic procedure.

Differential diagnosis

Many conditions cause localised pain or oedema on the lower extremities. Differential diagnosis of DVT includes cellulitis, lymphoedema, ruptured Baker's cyst, ruptured calf muscles/tendons and severe muscle cramps. History and examination are as important as invasive investigations.

Complications

PE is a serious and frequent complication of DVT. Pulmonary emboli are detected by perfusion lung scanning in approximately 50% of patients with documented DVT and asymptomatic DVT is found in 70% of patients with confirmed clinically symptomatic PE. Although DVT may begin frequently in the veins of the calf, it is only when the thrombosis extends above the knee that serious pulmonary embolism will occur.

Prophylaxis

The most effective way of decreasing morbidity and mortality from DVT and PE is to institute prophylaxis in patients at risk. There are two strategies for effective prevention:

- primary prevention in all patients with medium or high risk for DVT

- secondary prevention by screening patients with a medium or high risk with objective diagnostic tests

The second approach is expensive, time consuming and can be applied only to a limited number of patients. Broad application of effective methods of prevention has been shown to be more cost effective than selective, intensive surveillance. Safe and effective forms of prophylaxis are available for all patients at significant risk. Primary prophylaxis is cost effective.

20

Risk factors for venous thrombo-embolism

Background factors

- Age >40 years
- Moderate to morbid obesity
- Immobility (bed rest >4 days)
- Pregnancy

- Puerperium
- High dose oestrogens
- Previous DVT or PE
- Thrombophilia
  - deficiency of antithrombin III, protein C and S
  - activated protein C resistance
  - anti-phospholipid antibody
  - lupus anticoagulant
- Homocystinaemia

Disease or surgical procedure

- Trauma or surgery (especially of pelvis, hip and lower limb)
- Malignancy (especially pelvic or abdominal metastases)
- Heart failure
- Recent myocardial infarction
- Paralysis of lower limbs
- Severe infection
- Inflammatory bowel disease
- Nephrotic syndrome
- Polycythaemia
- Paraproteinaemia
- Paroxysmal nocturnal haemoglobinuria
- Behçet's disease

Prophylaxis is attempted by modulating activation of blood coagulation and preventing venous stasis (remember Virchow's triad of changes in the vessel wall, pattern of blood flow and constituents of blood).

The following approaches are of proven value:

- low dose subcutaneous heparin
- intermittent pneumatic compression of legs
- oral anticoagulants
- graduated compression stocking
- low molecular weight heparin

Anti-platelet agents (e.g. aspirin) are less effective for prevention of DVT.

Classification of risk of DVT and PE for hospital patients

Low risk (incidence of proximal vein thrombosis = 0.4%, fatal PE <0.2%)

- patients <40 years undergoing major surgery (>30 min) with no other risk factors

20

■ patients undergoing minor surgery (<30 min) with no other risk factors

■ patients with minor trauma or illness with no thrombophilia, or history of DVT or PE

Medium risk (incidence of proximal vein thrombosis = 2–4%, fatal PE = 0.2–0.5%)

■ major surgery in patients >40 years with one or more other risk factors

■ major acute medical illness (e.g. myocardial infarction)

■ major trauma

■ minor surgery, trauma or illness in patients with previous DVT, PE or thrombophilia

■ plaster cast immobilisation of the leg in patients with minor injury

High risk (incidence of proximal vein thrombosis = 10–20%, fatal PE = 1–5%)

■ fracture of or major orthopaedic surgery to the pelvis, hip or leg

■ major pelvic or abdominal surgery for cancer

■ major surgery, trauma or illness in patients with previous DVT, PE or thrombophilia

■ leg paralysis

■ critical ischaemia or major leg amputation

Prophylactic measures related to risk

Low risk	early ambulation graduated compression stockings
Medium risk	graduated compression stockings intermittent pneumatic calf compression during operation subcutaneous low dose unfractionated heparin (e.g. 5,000 i.u. 12 hourly, with 5,000 i.u. 2 h prior to surgery) no need to monitor APTT OR subcutaneous low molecular weight heparin (e.g. enoxaparin 20 mg once daily)
High risk	graduated compression shockings intermittent pneumatic calf compression during operation adjusted dose subcutaneous unfractionated heparin (at upper range of normal APTT) subcutaneous low molecular weight heparin (e.g. enoxaparin 40 mg once daily) adjusted moderate dose warfarin (initial dose the evening before surgery, with subsequent doses titrated to an INR of 2–3)

20

Differences between unfractionated and low molecular weight heparin

Heparin initiates anti-coagulation rapidly but has a short duration of action. It is now referred to as either standard or unfractionated heparin, to distinguish it from the low molecular weight heparins (e.g. enoxaparin, tinzaparin). Heparin acts as an anticoagulant by potentiating the action of antithrombin III which normally inactivates factors IXa, Xa, XIa and XIIa (see Chapter 8: Perioperative management of coagulation), and inhibits platelet aggregration.

In low dosage, heparin acts only on factor X to prevent its activation in hyper-coagulable states (e.g. postoperatively), without affecting platelet aggregation and hence the ability to form clot.

Low molecular weight heparin inhibits factor X only (specifically has anti-Xa activity), and thus causes less systemic anti-coagulation effects, with less effect on platelet function and longer half-life. It probably causes less haemorrhagic events than unfractionated heparin, but this is controversial.

Low molecular weight heparins are as effective and as safe as unfractionated heparin in the prevention of venous thrombo-embolism. In orthopaedic surgery prophylaxis they are probably more effective. They have a longer duration of action than unfractionated heparin, can be given as a once daily subcutaneous dose and the standard prophylactic regimen does not require APTT monitoring.

Treatment

Immediately after diagnosis of DVT, formal anti-coagulation treatment should begin to prevent local extension of the thrombus, prevent embolisation of the thrombus and (in certain circumstances such as large iliofemoral thrombosis) to accelerate fibrinolysis.

Anti-coagulation of thromboses below the knee is controversial. Bed rest is advised until full anti-coagulation is established. The patient can then be mobilised with an elasticated graduated pressure stocking. Heparin is usually continued for 48 h with warfarin therapy continuing for a further 3 months. Anticoagulants do not affect the thrombus already present and are purely a prophylactic measure to prevent PE. If there is thought to be a very high risk of embolism, or if anticoagulation is contraindicated (for example intracerebral or ongoing intestinal haemorrhage), an inferior vena cava filter can be placed by a radiologist. This mechanical sieve will catch large emboli passing from the lower limbs to the right side of the heart.

20

Key points

1. Prevention is better than cure.

2. All at risk patients should have prophylactic treatment.

3. An accurate preoperative history can identify those patients most at risk.

4. DVT is a risk for all patients, not just those in the perioperative period.

Further reading

Hirsh J and Hoak J. Management of deep vein thrombosis and pulmonary embolism. A statement for healthcare professionals. Council on Thrombosis (in consultation with the Council on Cardiovascular Radiology), American Heart Association. Circulation 1996; 93(12):2212–2245.

20

21

Postoperative nausea and vomiting

Pete Young

Patients rank pain, nausea and vomiting amongst their greatest perioperative concerns. Postoperative nausea and vomiting (PONV) is extremely distressing, prolongs hospitalisation and if severe, can cause fluid and electrolyte imbalance and disruption of the operative site. Depending on the patient group studied the incidence of postoperative nausea and vomiting is between 14% and 82%.

Physiology

Nausea and vomiting is primarily controlled and co-ordinated by the vomiting centre situated (diffusely) in the brainstem. The neurochemistry of the vomiting centre is probably not as simple as Figure 21.1 suggests, as 40 different neurotransmitters have been identified in this area of the brain.

Efferent impulses from the vomiting centre influence brainstem nuclei (e.g. vasomotor, respiratory and salivary) and pass to the gastrointestinal tract to produce the vomiting reflex.

Afferent impulses are shown in Figure 21.1.

Chemoreceptor trigger zone (CTZ) – a group of cells in a highly vascular area close to the area postrema on the floor of the fourth ventricle. The CTZ has a tonic influence on the vomiting centre. It lies partially outside the blood brain barrier and is therefore sensitive to systemic emetic stimuli. Opioid, dopamine (D_2) and 5-hydroxytryptamine$_3$ (5HT$_3$) receptors play a role in the activity of the CTZ.

Cerebral cortical afferent inputs account for the powerful psychological component of nausea.

Labyrinthine stimulation, mediated by the vestibular and cerebellar nuclei increases vomiting centre activity. This is at least partly a cholinergic pathway. The glossopharyngeal and vagus nerves also play a role.

21

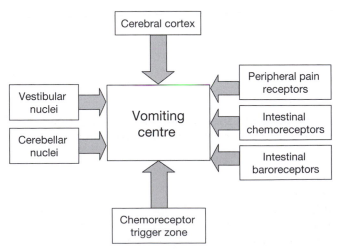

Fig. 21.1 The origins of the afferent neural inputs that influence nausea and vomiting.

Gut chemo- and baroreceptors and peripheral pain receptors all have direct effects on the vomiting centre.

Pharmacology

Antimuscarinic drugs

All drugs that cross the blood brain barrier and are muscarinic antagonists have anti-emetic properties. Centrally acting anti-cholinergic anti-emetics are most effective for motion sickness. Atropine, hyoscine and some anti-histaminergic (H_1) drugs are used. Hyoscine is more efficacious than atropine but is also more sedating. The sedative effects of centrally acting anti-cholinergic agents are probably due to suppression of the reticular activating system of the brainstem. Cyclizine has both anti-histaminergic and anti-cholinergic properties and is less sedating than hyoscine. It is also effective in suppressing the emetic effects of morphine.

Dopamine antagonists

Dopamine plays a key role at the CTZ and D_2 receptor antagonists are effective anti-emetics.

Phenothiazines

Phenothiazines generally have multiple pharmacological effects. Most have anti-muscarinic as well as anti-dopaminergic effects and many are also anti-histaminergic and antagonists at the 5HT receptors. Chlorpromazine is an effective antiemetic but causes sedation and extrapyramidal side effects. Thioridazine is less troublesome in this regard, but the most commonly used phenothiazine for PONV is prochlorperazine. It is less potent, but has a more acceptable side effect profile.

Butyrophenones

Haloperidol is a potent long acting antiemetic (a single dose lasts >24 h) but may be associated with extrapyramidal side effects. Droperidol has a shorter duration of action and is used in a low dosage for its anti-emetic properties. Some patients report feeling a disturbing inner anxiety with psychotic features, even with low doses of these agents.

21

Benzamides

At low doses, metoclopramide antagonises the D_2 receptor and at high doses it also has an effect at the $5HT_3$ receptor. Occasionally, extrapyramidal side effects occur at higher doses and especially in younger age groups. Metoclopramide also increases the rate of gastric emptying by peripheral dopaminergic mechanisms.

Domperidone

Domperidone has a similar action to metoclopramide, but does not cross the blood brain barrier and therefore does not cause dystonic reactions. For this reason it is useful in children.

5HT$_3$ receptor antagonists

Ondansetron, granisetron and tropisetron are potent selective 5HT$_3$ antagonists. Central effects occur at the CTZ and peripheral 5HT$_3$ receptors have been identified in the myenteric plexus of the intestinal wall. Ondansetron is commonly used as an anti-emetic with chemotherapy and is becoming increasingly popular perioperatively. They have a better side effect profile than many of the traditional agents and are at least as efficacious in PONV treatment and prevention.

Corticosteroids

Dexamethasone has been used as an anti-emetic during chemotherapy and has been used as a perioperative prophylactic although its place in PONV has yet to be established. The mode of action is uncertain.

The prevention and treatment of PONV

The aetiology of PONV is complex and multifactorial. There are patient, medical and surgical factors. The identification of patients at high risk of PONV is essential, in order to target prophylactic anti-emetic treatment.
   Risk factors include:

Patient factors

Past history of PONV	Young
Past history of motion sickness	Female sex

Surgical factors

Abdominal, gynaecological surgery	Long procedures
Squint and middle ear surgery	

Anaesthetic factors

Opioids	Anticholinesterases
Nitrous oxide	Premature post op oral fluids
Stormy induction (insufflation of gas to the stomach, hypoxic episodes)	
Other drugs, e.g. ergometrine	

21

A multi-modal approach to PONV

1. Combination therapy – using agents acting at different receptors (e.g. if prochlorperazine is inadequate add cyclizine, then add ondansetron in addition)

2. Use less emetogenic anaesthetic techniques (e.g. propofol infusions, avoidance of opioids using local anaesthesia techniques and/or NSAIDs)

3. Adequate intravenous hydration

4. Adequate pain control

Further reading

Gan TJ. Postoperative nausea and vomiting – can it be eliminated? JAMA 2002; 287(10): 1233–1236.

21

22

The management of perioperative pain

Parameswaran Pillai and Richard Neal

22

Pain is a conscious experience that incorporates sensory, cognitive, affective and behavioural components. Effective acute pain management reduces the incidence of postoperative complications and morbidity, reduces recovery time and increases patient satisfaction. Splinting of the diaphragm and poor cough due to abdominal or thoracic pain leads to lung atelectasis, retention of secretions and subsequent pneumonia. Release of stress hormones and catecholamines secondary to pain leads to increase in cardiac work and decreased intestinal motility, both of which can increase postoperative morbidity.

The key to effective pain management depends on:

- Knowledge of the anatomy and physiology of pain transmission

- Knowledge of the modes of action and side effects of analgesic drugs

- The ability to effectively assess pain severity

- An organised approach to prescribing

- Asking for help when pain management is not adequate

The pain pathways

The sense organs for pain are the naked nerve endings found in almost every tissue. Pain impulses are carried to the central nervous system (CNS) by two sets of fibres – small myelinated Aδ fibres carrying 'fast pain' and unmyelinated C fibres carrying 'slow pain'. Their cell bodies lie within the dorsal root ganglia and synapse with second order neurons in the dorsal horn of the spinal cord (Fig. 22.1). These neurons ascend in the contralateral spinothalamic and spinoreticular tracts to higher centres associated with consciousness, discrimination and affect (Fig. 22.2).

Inflammatory mediators such as prostaglandins, bradykinin and serotonin play an important role in sensitisation and activation of the nociceptors. They are released from the cell membrane debris of damaged cells.

Pain transmission can be modified at the dorsal horn by the descending Aβ fibres. They diminish transmission at this synapse by 'gating' it with inhibitory neurotransmitters such as GABA (gamma aminobutyric acid). Thus, higher cerebral centres are able to alter the intensity of pain sensation and these pathways provide further targets for pain treatment.

Methods of treating postoperative pain

- Pharmacological

  - Opioids

  - Non-steroidal anti-inflammatory drugs (NSAIDs) and related drugs

  - Local anaesthetics

  - Inhalational agents

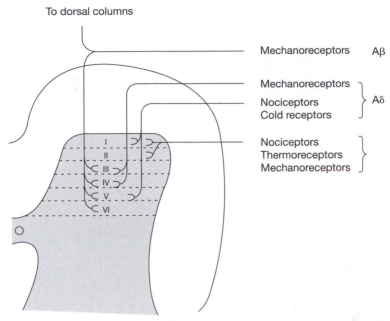

To dorsal columns

Mechanoreceptors   Aβ

Mechanoreceptors

Nociceptors   } Aδ
Cold receptors

Nociceptors
Thermoreceptors   }
Mechanoreceptors

Fig. 22.1 Schematic representation of the terminations of the three types of primary afferent neurons in the various layers of the dorsal horn of the spinal cord.

■ Non-pharmacological

   ● Cryotherapy

   ● Transcutaneous electrical nerve stimulation (TENS)

Modes of action and side effects of analgesic drugs

Opioids: Act by binding to specific opioid receptors; μ, κ and δ, thereby altering Ca^{2+} and K^+ conductance and intracellular cAMP (cyclic adenosine monophosphate) levels. This makes the cell membrane hyperpolarized and prevents transmission of action potentials. The μ-receptor mediates supraspinal analgesia, causes euphoria and physical dependence. Stimulation of the κ-receptor results in sedation, nausea and spinal analgesia.

Apart from analgesia, other effects of opioids include respiratory depression, sedation, cough suppression, vasodilatation, histamine release, nausea, tolerance, physical dependence and smooth muscle contraction caused by anti-cholinergic effects leading to constipation, miosis, biliary spasm, urinary retention, dry mouth and blurred vision.

Morphine remains the standard against which all other opioids are judged and is usually used as the first line treatment for severe pain. To administer a safe and effective dose of opioid, it should be carefully titrated to response.

22

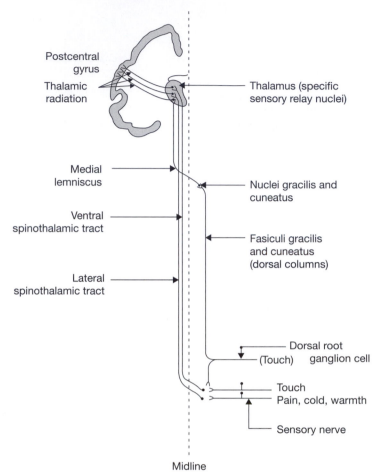

Postcentral gyrus

Thalamic radiation

Thalamus (specific sensory relay nuclei)

Medial lemniscus

Nuclei gracilis and cuneatus

Ventral spinothalamic tract

Fasiculi gracilis and cuneatus (dorsal columns)

Lateral spinothalamic tract

Dorsal root ganglion cell

(Touch)

Touch

Pain, cold, warmth

Sensory nerve

Midline

Fig. 22.2 Touch, pain and temperature pathways from the trunk and limbs. The anterolateral system (ventral and lateral spinothalamic and related ascending tracts) also projects to the mesencephalic reticular formation and the nonspecific thalamic nuclei.

There is no significant evidence to show that one opioid is better than another. The view that pethidine causes less smooth muscle constriction and is better for colicky and biliary pain has no good evidence base. When used in large quantities, accumulation of the metabolite norpethidine, a CNS irritant, may cause convulsions. Codeine (methylated morphine), has higher oral bioavailability and less potency compared to morphine. It causes less CNS and respiratory depression and is used as the first choice analgesic after intracranial neurosurgery. Tramadol is a weak opioid and has an inhibitory effect on neuronal uptake of noradrenaline (norepinephrine) and 5-hydroxytryptamine (5-HT) at CNS synapses. It causes less CNS and respiratory depression.

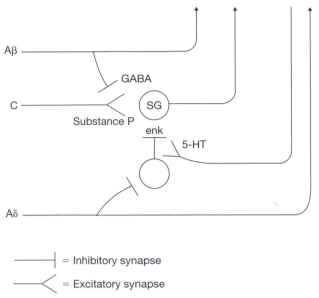

Aβ

GABA

C

SG

Substance P

enk

5-HT

Aδ

⊣ = Inhibitory synapse

< = Excitatory synapse

Fig. 22.3 Gate control theory of pain. enk, enkephalin; SG, substantia gelatinosa cell.

NSAIDs (Fig. 22.4): The analgesic action of NSAIDs results from inhibition of the enzyme cyclo-oxygenase (COX). Inhibition of the isoenzyme cyclo-oxygenase 2 decreases the synthesis of prostaglandins that stimulate the nociceptors. The side effects of the NSAIDs are attributed to the inhibition of cyclo-oxygenase 1, the constitutive isoenzyme that produces prostaglandins that regulate renal blood flow, platelet function and the production of the protective mucous layer in the gut wall. Specific COX-2 inhibitors like celecoxib and rofecoxib have been shown to decrease the incidence of gastrointestinal side effects, although none of them is strictly COX-2 selective, and whether they cause fewer renal side effects is debatable.

Young, brittle asthmatics with nasal polyps are at high risk of developing bronchoconstriction with NSAIDs. But if a patient with asthma has previously taken NSAIDs without incident, it is highly unlikely that they will be affected. Other contraindications to NSAID therapy include renal impairment, a recent gastrointestinal bleed or active gastric ulceration or coagulopathies. Care should be used in prescribing them to patients over the age of 65 years.

Paracetamol (acetaminophen): Paracetamol has central analgesic and antipyretic effects by mechanisms that are not yet fully understood. Even though it has effects similar to NSAIDs, it is not possible to demonstrate inhibition of cyclo-oxygenase with paracetamol *in vivo* or *in vitro*. It is effective for mild to moderate pain, is cheap, safe, well tolerated and is not a gastric irritant. It is however, very dangerous in overdose. As little as 5–7 g can produce fatal hepatic necrosis.

Local anaesthetic agents: Use of local anaesthetics in pain management is discussed elsewhere (see Chapter 18: Local anaesthetics). When assessing

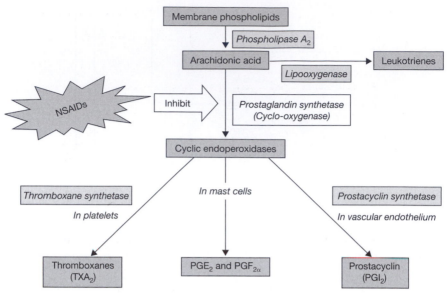

Fig. 22.4 The arachidonic acid pathway, and the inhibition of prostaglandin synthesis by NSAIDs.

a patient in pain, it should always be considered whether a local anaesthetic nerve block might be helpful.

Inhalational agents: The only agent currently in use is Entonox®, a mixture of 50% O_2 and 50% N_2O. When self administered by the patient it has a fast onset and a short duration of action that makes it an ideal analgesic for labour and painful procedures like dressing changes or the manipulation of dislocated joints. It can be used repeatedly and does not accumulate.

Cryotherapy: This involves the use of extreme cold to produce axonal degeneration without epineural or perineural damage, allowing slow regeneration. It can be applied perioperatively to intercostal nerves exposed during thoracotomy to provide prolonged postoperative analgesia. It has been associated with the development of neuromas.

Transcutaneous electrical nerve stimulation (TENS): Stimulation of peripheral nerves via cutaneous electrodes, to relieve pain. Its mechanism of action is based on the activation of descending, inhibitory fibres within the pain pathways, as described above in the gate theory of pain transmission (Fig. 22.3). TENS has been used with a varying degree of success in acute pain and chronic pain states. Its most common clinical use is in the relief of labour pain and chronic back pain.

Assessment of pain severity

Adequacy of analgesia and severity of side effects should be assessed frequently and appropriate alterations made. Medical and nursing staff

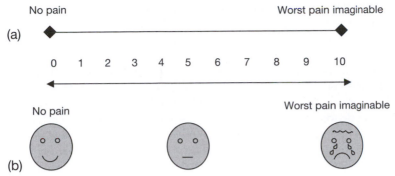

Fig. 22.5 Examples of visual analogue scales used by (a) adults and (b) children.

often underestimate the intensity of pain experienced by the patient. There is great individual variability between patients as to pain intensity when undergoing similar procedures. Some form of intensity rating scale should be used to score pain to have a subjective and systematic approach. Examples are given in Figure 22.5. Pain intensity should always be scored at rest and on movement. Assessment of pain intensity for a patient who is unable to communicate must be undertaken using an objective measure, rather than the pure subjectivity of the observer.

Pain intensity scoring
- Score out of 10. Ask the patient to score their pain out of 10, where zero is no pain, and ten is the worst pain imaginable.

- Linear analogue scale. Ask the patient to place a mark on a 10 cm line to indicate the severity of pain (Fig. 22.5a).

- Modified linear analogue scales for children (Fig. 22.5b).

- Complex pain questionnaires, e.g. Minnesota multiphasic personality inventory, more suited to chronic pain states.

Considerations when prescribing analgesics for postoperative pain

Preemptive analgesia is the concept of suppression of dorsal horn neuronal activity involved in pain pathways before a painful stimulus, in order to reduce analgesic requirements postoperatively. Techniques include central neuronal blockade, local anaesthetic infiltration and use of NSAIDs and opioids.

Balanced analgesia is the use of a combination of drugs and techniques to achieve adequate analgesia. Each drug reduces the requirement for the others, thereby reducing the side effects caused by any single agent. This is particularly important for opioids. If opioids were prescribed alone for

22

severe pain, patients would experience many of the side effects without necessarily being free of pain. When combined with regular paracetamol and an NSAID, analgesia is better and both the dose of opioid and side effects are reduced.

This concept can be explained because there are two components to perioperative pain. **Background** pain is a constant pain related to the pathology or wound, which is best treated using regular analgesia with long-acting drugs. **Breakthrough** pain is additional acute exacerbation of pain caused by movement and is controlled by drugs with rapid onset and short duration of action. The route of administration chosen also influences the time of onset and length of action of the chosen analgesics. The advantages and disadvantages of different routes of administration are summarised in Figure 22.6.

Route	Advantages	Disadvantages
Oral	Easy. Preferred by patients. 'Slow-release' preparations may be available to extend duration of action. Best suited to providing drugs to treat background pain.	Unsuitable in patients who are uncooperative, strictly 'nil by mouth', are vomiting profusely or have ileus. Most orally administered drugs are absorbed slowly. Unpredictable absorption due to degradation by stomach acid and enzymes.
Rectal	Good absorption – the inferior haemorrhoidal veins drain directly into the inferior vena cava, avoiding hepatic "first pass" metabolism. Well suited for administration of analgesics for background pain.	May not be suitable after rectal or anal surgery. Some patients dislike suppositories.
Subcutaneous or intramuscular	Good absorption, especially for drugs that are broken down in the gut, are poorly or unpredictably absorbed or are extensively metabolised by the liver (e.g. morphine). Onset more rapid than the above routes – drugs for breakthrough pain can be administered this way.	Absorption may still be unpredictable if peripheries are poorly perfused. Hurts, causes bruising and frightens children and needle phobics. Duration of action varies depending on drug preparation.

Intravenous	Dependable and reproducible effects. Entire administered dose reaches the systemic circulation immediately – the dose can be accurately titrated against response. Ideal for treating breakthrough pain.	Requires a functioning cannula. More expensive and labour intensive than other routes. Cannulation is distressing to some patients, especially children. Cannulae are prone to infection. IV injection of drugs may cause local reactions. Needs close supervision. Risk of overdose.
Topical	Easy. Non-invasive. High levels of patient satisfaction.	Most drugs have a high molecular weight and are poorly lipid soluble so are not absorbed via skin or mucous membranes. Fentanyl can be given as a patch or lollipop. Very slow absorption – suitable for background analgesia only.
Inhaled	Very rapid absorption due to the huge surface area of the respiratory endothelium.	The only analgesic currently administered by inhalation is N_2O, as Entonox ®
Epidural	Analgesia can be targeted to specific anatomical regions, such as a series of dermatomes. Opioid sparing. Lower incidence of DVT. Allows coughing and decreases incidence of pulmonary morbidity after major abdominal surgery. Allows early mobilisation after hip or knee surgery.	Requires expertise of anaesthetists/acute pain team. High levels of monitoring and nursing input on the ward. Hypotension. 1% incidence of postdural puncture headache. Rare but devastating side effects of epidural abscess or haematoma.

Fig. 22.6 The advantages and disadvantages of giving drugs by different routes.

Patients who are already taking opioids require a different approach that may involve alternative classes of drugs or regional analgesia. Specialist help should be sought early in these cases.

22

Anti-emetic therapy (see Chapter 21: Postoperative nausea and vomiting) and aperients (e.g. senna or lactulose) should be considered if opioids are given.

Intravenous patient-controlled analgesia (PCA) is a system of opioid delivery that consists of an infusion pump incorporating a timing device. The patient can titrate the analgesic dose required for optimal control of pain. The patient presses a button to deliver a preset low dose of opioid, most commonly morphine. A preset lock out period then follows which prevents over dosage. It is suited to treat breakthrough pain and to some extent background pain as well. A background infusion may be added, but this increases the risk of respiratory depression. Patients on PCA regimes require a higher level of monitoring. Respiratory rate and level of consciousness should be monitored to guard against the onset of respiratory depression. PCA requires intravenous access and is not suitable for patients who cannot understand how to use the machine or are physically incapable of pressing the button.

Asking for help: Many hospitals have established multidisciplinary acute pain teams consisting of nurses and anaesthetists. These teams counsel patients preoperatively who require specialist pain management techniques such as PCA and epidurals, and monitor the patients and manage these devices postoperatively. They also take referrals of other acute pain problems in the hospital.

Key points

- Analgesic prescriptions should have a good evidence base and prescribing guidelines should be agreed using a multidisciplinary approach, involving anaesthetists, surgeons, nurses and pharmacists, in order to simplify prescribing for junior medical staff. Standards for pain management should also be set allowing for better auditing of practice and to identify ongoing clinical and educational needs. Acute Pain Services have done much to further educational and clinical support of postoperative pain management, for both patients and health care professionals.

- Education of all health care professionals and patients remains the key to effective pain management. Adequate knowledge will dispel the myths and misconceptions that continue to afflict the provision of adequate and effective postoperative analgesia.

Further reading

Besson JM. The neurobiology of pain. Lancet 1999; 353:1610.

Brian Ready L. Acute Perioperative Pain. In: Ronald D. Miller (ed.). Anesthesia. 5th edn. Churchill Livingstone, 2000, p 2323.

Guidelines for the Use of Non-steroidal Anti-inflammatory Drugs in the Perioperative Period. 1998. The Royal College of Anaesthetists. London. (this document, others and useful links can be obtained from www.rcoa.ac.uk)

Power I and Smith G. Postoperative Pain. In: Alan R. Aitkenhead, David J. Rowbotham and Graham Smith (eds). Textbook of Anaesthesia. 4th edn. Churchill Livingstone, 2001, p 544.

22

23

High dependency and recovery units

Helen Smith

23

The postoperative period is a very important time for any patient, from those undergoing routine uncomplicated surgery and anaesthesia (including day surgery), to those who are critically ill. Requirements are for close monitoring of the patient by staff proficient in airway maintenance and the recognition and management of anaesthetic and surgical complications. The recovery unit staff aim to discharge the patient with any pain or nausea/vomiting under control and with the patient well hydrated with provision for further fluids and analgesia as required. The patient should be alert, orientated with stable vital signs and any complications recognised and treated.

The services offered by the recovery and high dependency unit (HDU) are basically the same. The HDU has the capacity for an extended recovery with greater and more intense provision of nursing care for longer periods, caring for sicker patients who need more invasive monitoring or specialised analgesic techniques (e.g. epidurals). The HDU would not normally accept patients requiring mechanical ventilation. The HDU in some hospitals also admits non-surgical patients. Such patients often have single organ failure. If such disease is severe, or there is more than one organ system affected, admission to intensive care may be more appropriate. The HDU centralises skilled nursing staff and expensive equipment, such as monitoring and drug infusion devices. Centralising acutely ill patients also simplifies medical supervision, especially out of hours.

Need for immediate access to anaesthetic assistance

The medical supervision and co-ordination of patient care is the responsibility of the anaesthetist. An anaesthetist should always be immediately available for the management of postoperative complications and cardiopulmonary resuscitation. The discharge of the patient from recovery remains the responsibility of the anaesthetist.

Monitors
The most important monitor is the presence of the recovery nurse with anaesthetic backup. Pulse oximetry, non-invasive blood pressure, ECG, temperature, pain and sedation scores are the basic monitoring requirements with the ability to measure invasive blood pressure and central venous pressure if required. Fluid balance should be monitored with particular emphasis on urine output.

Respiratory complications

1. Airway obstruction
The most common cause of airway obstruction in the supine unconscious patient is the sagging of the tongue backwards into the oropharynx.

This can be overcome in most patients by simple airway manoeuvres (such as chin lift or jaw thrust) which bring the tongue forward, away from the back of the oropharynx. The recovery position benefits the patient by drawing the tongue forward. It also is the best possible position for a patient who is vomiting or regurgitating as the vomitus will drain out of the mouth rather than into the lungs. Every bed or trolley in the recovery room should have the ability to tip the patient head down – essential if the patient is vomiting or bleeding from the airway to prevent aspiration.

If forward movement of the mandible is insufficient, an oral or nasal airway can help open the airway (a conscious patient will gag on an oral airway). Sometimes a patient will require assistance with ventilation using a mask with a self-inflating bag attached to an oxygen supply (up to ~90% oxygen can be administered in this way). A foreign body can also cause upper airway obstruction. Dentures should have been removed before the operation. There have been some fatalities following failure to remove throat packs postoperatively.

Laryngeal spasm can occur in the postoperative period particularly if mucus, blood or secretions are irritating the vocal cords. Initially this can be dealt with by applying 100% oxygen to the patient with continuous positive airway pressure (CPAP) given by hand. Sometimes suction of the oropharynx is required. If the patient does not respond by opening the airway with these manoeuvres then tracheal intubation with prior administration of a muscle relaxant is required.

2. Hypoxaemia

This is a relatively common and potentially serious postoperative complication. This can be caused by:

- Low inspired oxygen

- Areas of low ventilation/perfusion (V/Q) ratio

- Right to left shunt

- Hypoventilation

All patients recovering from general anaesthesia should be given supplemental oxygen.

The most common cause of postoperative hypoxaemia is an increase in the right-to-left pulmonary shunt. If an alveolus collapses, due to atelectasis (blockage with secretions, blood or infected matter) or pressure from without (decreased functional residual capacity), it will still be perfused with pulmonary capillary blood. Alveoli that are perfused but not ventilated cannot contribute to gas exchange, so blood with a haemoglobin saturation more appropriate for the venous circulation enters the left ventricle and is pumped around the body causing hypoxaemia. After anaesthesia, and especially after major abdominal or thoracic surgery, functional residual capacity is reduced so alveolar collapse is more of a problem. Neonates, the obese and women in the third trimester of pregnancy already have a reduced functional residual capacity so are even more prone to shunt and hypoxia.

Pneumothorax can occur as a result of direct lung or airway injury from trauma or attempts at central venous cannulation or as a complication of artificial ventilation with high inflation pressures. This causes hypoxaemia due to both atelectasis and intrapulmonary shunt. If a patient with a pneumothorax is mechanically ventilated, or has a pneumothorax of >20%, a chest drain should be inserted.

Pulmonary oedema is another cause of postoperative hypoxaemia due to high hydrostatic pressure in the pulmonary capillaries, an increased capillary permeability or following sustained reductions in the interstitial hydrostatic pressure. Treatment includes diuretics, fluid restriction and vasodilators. Positive pressure ventilation is useful if there is severe hypoxaemia or respiratory acidosis.

An increased metabolic rate can make hypoxaemia worse. If a patient is shivering, hyperthermic or a small child, the metabolic rate is much higher and hypoxaemia develops sooner. (see Chapter 24: Postoperative hypoxia)

3. Hypoventilation

The most common cause of hypoventilation is the residual effect of drugs administered intra-operatively. Central respiratory depression is seen with any general anaesthetic. The effect is often exacerbated by the use of opioids given for pain relief. All opioid analgesics produce a dose dependent depression of respiration with the elderly being particularly sensitive.

Poor respiratory muscle function occurs following surgery and often contributes to hypoventilation. Patients undergoing upper abdominal surgery have the greatest reduction in vital capacity particularly if the patient is in pain. This leads to problems with both carbon dioxide elimination and oxygenation. Obesity, abdominal distension and tight dressings also inhibit respiratory muscle function and can predispose to CO_2 retention.

Circulatory complications

1. Hypotension

Hypotension in the recovery phase of anaesthesia is usually due to decreased ventricular preload, reduced myocardial contractility or a profound decrease in systemic vascular resistance.

■ Hypovolaemia
A reduced ventricular preload may result from inadequately replaced fluid losses or postoperative bleeding. Bleeding into surgical drains or wounds will provide an obvious guide to losses. However, concealed intra-abdominal or retroperitoneal fluid losses may occur. There may also

be unmeasured (so called insensible) losses by sweating and exposure. The former is a significant problem in pyrexia. Diagnosis is dependent on the presence of impaired circulation with hypotension and failure of a sustained response to fluid challenge. The usual cause of postoperative bleeding is inadequate surgical haemostasis but coagulation abnormalities also need to be considered. Hypovolaemia may also be caused by the sympathetic block associated with spinal or epidural anaesthesia. The signs of hypovolaemia are tachycardia, low blood pressure, poor capillary refill, low urine output and low central venous pressure (CVP). Treatment should include replacement of the fluids lost, administration of oxygen and surgical haemostasis.

23

■ Cardiogenic shock
Failure of the left ventricle causing hypotension results most frequently from perioperative myocardial infarction (MI) or over-transfusion, and may lead to pulmonary oedema and respiratory distress. The ECG should be monitored and cardiac enzymes estimated to exclude an MI (although a diagnostic rise is not seen for several hours). Treatment includes oxygen, fluid restriction and diuretics. Inotropic support may be necessary in some cases. If there is co-existant right heart failure, the jugulovenous pressure or CVP will be elevated.

■ Septic shock
Hypotension due to a reduction in the systemic vascular resistance despite an increase in cardiac output is frequently caused by bacterial lipopolysaccharide or the pro-inflammatory cytokines released in sepsis. Fluid resuscitation and inotropic support is often required along with appropriate antibiotic cover (see Chapter 25: Postoperative hypotension), and invasive monitoring on ICU.

2. Hypertension
The commonest cause of postoperative hypertension is pain. Other causes include inadequately treated preoperative hypertension, hypoxia, hypercapnia, over-transfusion, a full bladder and the use of vasopressor drugs. The cause needs to be identified quickly and treated appropriately. Hypertension increases cardiac work and myocardial oxygen consumption and can lead to left ventricular failure and myocardial infarction.

3. Arrhythmias
These are frequently seen in the recovery area and are often benign. Those leading to cardiovascular instability need investigating and treating. The common causes are pain, hypoxia, hypercapnia, electrolyte and acid/base disturbances and myocardial ischaemia.

Conscious level
Postoperative unconsciousness is usually ascribed to anaesthetic agents but other causes need to be considered especially if there is no improvement

or even a deterioration in the conscious level. Blood sugar levels should be checked for the possibility of hypoglycaemia. Other causes include hypercapnia, hypotension and hypothermia. Cerebral insults such as intra-operative cerebrovascular accident, intracranial bleed or epilepsy should also be considered.

Analgesia

A wide range of analgesics is used. Pain can be the cause of patient agitation, hypertension, cardiac arrhythmias, respiratory insufficiency as well as discomfort for the patient.

Analgesic requirements and techniques should be discussed with the patient preoperatively. Many patients are given non-steroidal anti-inflammatory (NSAIDs) drugs as premedication or at induction of anaesthesia. Intra-operatively a combination of long and short-acting intravenous opioids is used, often with peripheral or central neural blockade. All such modes of analgesia can be continued into the postoperative period.

Patient controlled analgesia (PCA) with an intravenous opioid such as morphine and epidural infusions (e.g. bupivacaine and fentanyl) can be used to control severe pain for several days. Epidurals need specialised nursing care and need to be utilised only in areas where nurses are trained to deal with the complications. Simple analgesics such as paracetamol and NSAIDs can be used in combination with opioids. The rationale behind using 'combination therapy' is that the simple analgesics have an 'opioid sparing' effect, thereby decreasing the side effects of the opioid analgesics (especially sedation and nausea/vomiting). (see Chapter 22: Management of perioperative pain)

Management of nausea and vomiting

Nausea and vomiting are very frequent complications and can lead to patient discomfort and prolonged stay in the recovery unit. The cause depends on many factors including patient susceptibility, type of operation and anaesthetic technique. Anti-emetics are frequently given preoperatively or at induction. Research and audit suggest that anti-emetics are better at prevention than treatment. (see Chapter 21: Postoperative nausea and vomiting)

Communication is essential

The anaesthetist, theatre staff and surgeon have a responsibility to communicate as comprehensively as possible to recovery staff details of:

- Patient's premorbid state

- Drug history and allergies

- Intra-operative procedure

- Intra-operative complications

- Any anticipated complications

- Analgesic and fluid requirements

The recovery nurses need to pass this information on to the ward staff when the patient is discharged from the recovery area.

Special considerations

Day surgery

The other important issues relating to patient recovery are the discharge criteria for patients undergoing day surgery, as these patients do not have the luxury of immediate medical input. Day surgery units have strict policies to ensure that patients with ongoing or developing postoperative complications are not discharged inappropriately. The discharge criteria need to be equally as stringent regarding the written information given to each patient and the responsible adult accompanying them home. Such information should outline what each patient might expect and who to contact if concerns are raised.

Paediatrics

Ideally children should be dealt with in a separate child-orientated environment with paediatric-trained staff and play nurses. As has been stated by many, children are not just small adults. The profile of problems postoperatively is very different from the adult population. Laryngeal reflexes are prominent and laryngospasm is far easier to induce. Children primarily respond to hypoxaemia by a fall in heart rate. Encouraging parents to attend the recovery room is not widespread but is increasingly seen as meeting the psychological needs of the children.

Further reading

Immediate Postanaesthetic Recovery. Association of Anaesthetists of Great Britain and Ireland, 2002. www.aagbi.org

23

24

Postoperative hypoxia

Mark Abrahams

Aetiology, assessment and management

Every cell utilises oxygen in metabolism to provide the energy necessary for the processes and functions essential for life. Our respiratory and circulatory systems are designed for the purpose of transporting atmospheric oxygen to the body tissues. Hypoxia occurs when oxygen delivery to the tissues fails to meet the metabolic demand and results in impaired cellular function and an increase in anaerobic metabolism leading to intracellular acidosis, further impairment in cellular function and eventual organ failure.

There are four main classifications of hypoxia:

1. **Hypoxic hypoxia**: The arterial blood being pumped to the tissues has reduced levels of dissolved oxygen (a low oxygen tension or partial pressure of oxygen – P_aO_2). This is known as hypoxaemia, and implies a failure of gas exchange between alveoli and pulmonary capillaries.

2. **Anaemic hypoxia**: Most of the oxygen in the blood is transported to peripheral tissues in red blood cells as oxyhaemoglobin. Anaemia or carbon monoxide poisoning will reduce the ability of blood to carry oxygen.

3. **Circulatory hypoxia**: The body requires a functioning circulatory system to carry oxygenated blood to the tissues that require it. Failure of the circulation globally (e.g. in severe shock or cardiac arrest) or locally (e.g. in arterial thrombosis) will lead to tissue hypoxia.

4. **Histotoxic hypoxia**: The tissue cells are unable to utilise the delivered oxygen. This can occur in some toxicity states, e.g. cyanide poisoning.

Any of the above may potentially cause hypoxia in the postoperative patient.

The postoperative patient

In the healthy body, homeostatic systems work together efficiently to ensure that tissue demand for oxygen is met with adequate supply, and tissue hypoxia will only occur during times of unusual stress (e.g. heavy exercise). Disease states however, are frequently associated with reduced oxygen supply locally (e.g. coronary artery disease) or globally (e.g. respiratory failure). After surgery, the stress response to injury (catecholamines, cortisol), infection and healing combine to increase tissue oxygen demand. The function of the perioperative physician can be distilled into one aim: to ensure that oxygen supply meets oxygen demand.

Increased oxygen demand in the postoperative patient

A healthy conscious resting adult will normally utilise approximately 250 ml of oxygen per minute. The postoperative patient however, may have a much greater demand for oxygen due to the following reasons:

- Underlying disease state: patients undergoing operations frequently have underlying illnesses that lead to increased metabolic requirement.

- Tissue healing and stress response: the stress response following tissue injury leads to stimulation of inflammatory and tissue repair processes.

- Increased cardiac work: the release of stress hormones and vasoactive substances associated with tissue injury and pain and the fluid shifts occurring during major operations, will increase the work of the heart. The increased sympathetic response related to the re-establishment of REM (rapid eye movement) sleep is thought to account for an increase in morbidity occurring on the second or third postoperative night. This is the basis for using supplementary oxygen therapy at night for at-risk postoperative patients.

- Immunological response: any disruption of the skin or protective membranes will expose the patient to the risk of invasion by infective organisms. The body's immunological defences will be stimulated following surgery.

24

Decreased oxygen supply in the postoperative patient

Impaired oxygen supply is almost universal in postoperative patients and is due to a breakdown in the delivery of oxygen from the atmosphere to the peripheral tissues that need it. The severity of hypoxia in the postoperative patient depends upon surgical, anaesthetic, medical, physiological and pharmacological considerations, leading to impairment of those systems responsible for oxygen transport. (See 'Causes of postoperative hypoxia')

Assessment and management of the hypoxic postoperative patient

1. Take a brief history.

2. Give the patient oxygen via a mask with reservoir bag to deliver as high a concentration as possible. There is no place for low-concentration oxygen delivery systems in acutely hypoxic patients. (Only a very small percentage of patients with chronic obstructive pulmonary disease will rely upon their hypoxic drive to maintain adequate ventilation.) Monitor the effectiveness of supplementary oxygen with a peripheral oxygen saturation probe. Regular arterial blood gas samples may need to be taken. Sit the patient upright if conscious, normotensive and if the surgery allows.

3. Call for senior help if necessary.

4. Assessment of any sick patient should always begin with the ABCs: Airway, Breathing and Circulation.

- **Assess the airway**: Look and feel for signs of obstruction of the upper airways. Listen for stridor. If the patient is unable to maintain an adequate airway, try simple manoeuvres such as chin lift or jaw thrust. If unsuccessful consider inserting a nasal or oro-pharyngeal (Guedel) airway. In the event of continuing difficulties, call for anaesthetic help immediately.

- **Assess breathing**: Measure the respiratory rate. Examine for signs of hypoxia or carbon dioxide retention, including central cyanosis, the use of accessory muscles of respiration and flapping tremor. Look and feel for uneven or inadequate ventilation, altered patterns of respiration, tracheal deviation and signs of respiratory distress. Auscultate the chest for added or absent sounds. In particular, postoperative patients are at risk of aspiration pneumonia, pulmonary oedema, atelectasis, lung collapse, pneumothorax, haemothorax, pulmonary thromboembolism, fat embolism and ARDS (acute respiratory distress syndrome).

- **Assess circulation**: Feel the pulse rate, rhythm and volume. Look for adequacy of peripheral circulation and assess skin temperature. Check non-invasive blood pressure and jugular venous pulse (or CVP if available). Check for pulsus paradoxus. Examine oral membranes for signs of cyanosis or dehydration and conjunctiva for signs suggesting anaemia. Examine the praecordium, noting significant or new murmurs or heart sounds. Auscultate for signs of pulmonary oedema, feel for an enlarged liver and assess peripheral oedema. Examine legs for signs of deep venous thrombosis. Monitor hourly urine output.

5. Assess neurological status, noting conscious level, size and reactivity of pupils. Hypoventilation due to opioid analgesics is a common cause of postoperative hypoxia.

6. Examine the abdomen looking for distension leading to impairment of diaphragmatic function, and the possibility of intra-abdominal haemorrhage.

7. **Warm patient**: Aim for a core temperature of 36–37°C. Shivering increases oxygen requirements.

8. Investigations should initially include full blood count, urea and electrolytes, arterial blood gases, ECG and chest X-ray. Continuous pulse oximetry is essential for adequate monitoring of the patient with hypoxia or at risk of hypoxia.

9. Treat the cause of the hypoxia appropriately (see page 203).

10. Reassess, complete the secondary survey of the patient, treating any abnormalities appropriately.

11. Ensure adequate surgical analgesia. A patient in pain will not breathe adequately, particularly if the operation site is thoracic or upper

abdominal. In addition, if the patient is unable to move or cough because of pain, he is at greater risk of morbidity due to respiratory infection.

12. Consider further treatment modalities including physiotherapy.

13. Consider the need for ventilatory support. Continued respiratory insufficiency may necessitate the use of invasive ventilation techniques.

Causes of postoperative hypoxia

The following lists the more common causes of hypoxia in the postoperative ward patient.

a. Surgical causes

■ **Pain**: Inadequate analgesia following surgery may cause pain on respiration and coughing, especially with thoracic or upper abdominal operations. The patient in pain has an increased risk of hypoxia due to hypoventilation, atelectasis and respiratory infection.

■ **Hypovolaemic shock**: Due to inadequate fluid resuscitation or continuing blood loss.

■ **Anaesthesia**: Basal atelectasis, lung collapse, aspiration of stomach or oropharyngeal contents and aspiration of blood are all potential complications of general anaesthesia and can contribute to hypoxia in the postoperative period. (See Anaesthetic agents below.) Hypothermia can lead to shivering with subsequently increased oxygen requirements.

■ **Pneumothorax**: Due to central venous line insertion or thoracic surgery, but can occur spontaneously or with positive pressure ventilation during anaesthesia.

■ **Abdominal distension**: Blood, gas or fluid can cause abdominal distension leading to diaphragmatic splinting, hypoventilation and basal atelectasis.

■ **Neuromuscular injury**: Phrenic, recurrent laryngeal or intercostal nerve damage or direct trauma to the structures and muscles of respiration.

b. Pharmacological causes

■ **Anaesthetic agents**: Respiratory depression, alteration in lung ventilation/perfusion matching and hypoxia due to the diffusion properties of nitrous oxide can all occur in the operative and immediate postoperative periods. These effects, however, are short lasting and unlikely to be causes of hypoxia in the surgical ward.

■ **Opioid analgesics**: Respiratory depression due to opioid overdose is a common cause of hypoxia in the postoperative patient, particularly in the elderly.

■ **Sedative agents**: Benzodiazepines and other sedative agents can cause respiratory depression. Again, elderly patients are at particular risk.

24

c. Acute medical conditions

■ **Cardiac failure**: This has multiple causes, including fluid overload, myocardial infarction, drug toxicity, etc. Cardiogenic shock will cause circulatory hypoxia whereas left ventricular failure and subsequent pulmonary oedema will disrupt oxygen diffusion in the lungs.

■ **Respiratory infection**

■ **Bronchospasm**

■ **Pulmonary thromboembolism**: Effectively reduces perfusion to a section of lung, and causes shunt and cardiac dysrhythmias.

■ **Gas embolism**: May be iatrogenic (e.g. unclamped lumen on central venous cannula). Complication of surgery to the head and neck or after shoulder surgery.

■ **Fat embolism**: Prevalent following surgery for long bone fractures in patients suffering a major trauma.

■ **Acute respiratory distress syndrome**: Complication of major traumatic insult to the body, including massive blood transfusion, sepsis, major trauma, shock, etc.

■ **Sepsis**: Poor tissue perfusion due to septic shock will lead to tissue hypoxia.

■ Consider other medical causes including cardiac tamponade, tracheo-bronchial obstruction and pleural effusion.

An overview of pulse oximetry

Most of the oxygen in arterial blood is carried in the red blood cells as oxyhaemoglobin. Each fully saturated haemoglobin molecule carries 4 oxygen molecules and is designed to release the oxygen when exposed to a high oxygen diffusion gradient. The oxyhaemoglobin molecule changes shape as it releases a molecule of oxygen, making the subsequent release of oxygen molecules easier, and giving rise to the sigmoid shape of the oxyhaemoglobin saturation curve (see next page). Thus, oxyhaemoglobin retains its oxygen molecules in areas with high ambient oxygen tension (e.g. as the oxygenated blood leaves the lungs), but can release them quickly when exposed to environments with low ambient oxygen tension (e.g. ischaemic tissue).

The change in shape of the haemoglobin molecule with the level of oxygenation alters its ability to absorb different wavelengths of light, giving rise to the red and blue colours of oxygenated and deoxygenated haemoglobin respectively. The pulse oximeter exploits these differences by measuring the absorption of different wavelengths of light, calculating the ratio of deoxyhaemoglobin to oxyhaemoglobin in arterial blood

24

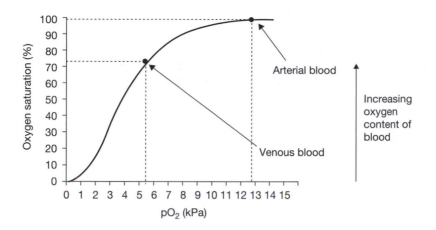

24

(by isolating pulsatile flow), and giving this ratio as a percentage of fully oxygenated (fully saturated) blood.

Since most of the oxygen in blood is carried in combination with the haemoglobin molecule, the oxygen saturation gives an accurate indication of the oxygen content of arterial blood, providing the patient's haemoglobin concentration is normal. (An anaemic patient's arterial blood, though fully saturated, will carry less oxygen!) Oxygen saturation levels above 90% are associated with high oxygen content and the pulse oximeter is most accurate above this level. Below 90%, small drops in ambient oxygen tension precipitate large drops in the oxygen content of arterial blood (the steep section of the oxyhaemoglobin dissociation curve) and may lead to tissue hypoxia.

The pulse oximeter requires pulsatile blood flow to isolate arterial oxygen saturation and is less effective when used on patients with poor peripheral circulation, e.g. hypotension, vasoconstriction or with irregular arterial pulsation, e.g. atrial fibrillation. In addition, the performance of the pulse oximeter may be affected by nail varnish or dirt staining on fingers, by optical interference due to external light sources and by interference due to abnormal haemoglobins, e.g. carbon monoxide poisoning and smoking. (see Chapter 19: Monitoring used in the perioperative period)

25

Postoperative hypotension

Chris Sharpe

Postoperative hypotension is a common occurrence, and has many causes. It may be defined as a systolic blood pressure of less than 70 mmHg. Patients with cardiovascular disease, the elderly and those undergoing major surgery are very susceptible to hypotension and this can be detrimental. It can result in a lengthened hospital stay due to increased morbidity and if left untreated may result in organ dysfunction, with subsequent organ system failure, e.g. myocardial infarction, cerebrovascular accident, renal failure and death.

Basic treatment consists of oxygen therapy, lying the patient flat and treatment of the underlying cause.

Mean arterial blood pressure is governed by the formula:

$$MABP = CO \times SVR$$

Therefore hypotension may be due to factors causing a reduced cardiac output (CO) or a low systemic vascular resistance (SVR).

Factors reducing cardiac output

Hypovolaemia

Hypovolaemia is the most common cause of postoperative hypotension. This may be due to:

1. Inadequate intra-operative fluid replacement.

2. Ongoing haemorrhage. Observe the operative site, any increased flow through the drains, a falling CVP despite fluid replacement or overt bleeding.

3. Fluid shifts into the transcellular ('third') space, e.g. after major abdominal surgery.

4. Large volume nasogastric losses.

5. Large unmeasured 'insensible' losses, e.g. pyrexia.

These losses must be replaced with the appropriate fluid. Most doctors are overcautious about prescribing fluids for fear of precipitating cardiac failure. For this reason, nearly all patients, especially the elderly or those with a history of ischaemic heart disease, are denied sufficient fluid. These groups of patients are, in fact, most reliant on maintaining adequate ventricular filling pressures and coronary perfusion. A strategy akin to that on page 48 should be adopted to ensure optimal fluid management. Glucose saline or 5% glucose are not appropriate resuscitation fluids as the intravascular half life is very short. These hypotonic solutions may cause hyponatraemia. (see Chapter 6: Perioperative management of emergency surgery and Chapter 7: Perioperative fluid management)

Left ventricular failure

This may occur in the postoperative period as a result of myocardial ischaemia or as a result of over transfusion with fluids. Features suggestive of this condition include cold extremities, dyspnoea, elevated jugular venous or central venous pressure and basal crepitations on auscultation of the chest. Treatment includes reducing fluid infusion rates, oxygen therapy and diuretics. A positive inotropic agent may be indicated.

Cardiac rhythm

Cardiac arrhythmias may be associated with hypotension. Those that may be seen in the postoperative period include fast atrial fibrillation, supraventricular tachycardias and ventricular tachycardia. As diastolic filling time is affected more by the heart rate than systole, the faster the rate the less the ventricles fill with blood resulting in a low cardiac output. Patients with these arrhythmias require cardiac monitoring and correction of the arrhythmia using anti-arrhythmic drugs. However if the patient is significantly compromised then cardioversion may be necessary to convert the patient back to sinus rhythm. Atrial fibrillation is one of the more common arrhythmias, characterised by an irregularly irregular pulse. Hypotension associated with this rhythm is made worse due to the lack of the atrial systolic component in ventricular filling during late diastole. Always remember to check electrolytes as electrolyte imbalance may contribute to these arrhythmias and therefore must be corrected. Hypokalaemia and hypomagnesaemia are very important in this respect.

25

Drugs

The effect of drugs should be considered as a cause of hypotension. Antihypertensives are a common contributor especially β-blockers, calcium channel blockers, and angiotensin converting enzyme inhibitors. β-blockers are notorious for hypotension as they abolish the normal compensatory mechanisms to hypotension.

Obstruction

Obstruction includes cardiac tamponade, tension pneumothorax and embolism. Each of these must be differentiated using history and examination. For example, hypotension with dyspnoea after insertion of a central venous catheter suggests a tension pneumothorax. This is life threatening and will require immediate decompression by inserting a needle (cannula) in the second intercostal space on the affected side in the mid-clavicular line. This must then be followed by the insertion of a definitive chest drain. Embolism may be pulmonary (associated with dyspnoea and history of immobility, obesity, orthopaedic or gynaecological surgery), or it may be fat (long bone fractures) and require specific treatment.

Factors affecting the systemic vascular resistance

Residual effects of anaesthetic drugs

Nearly all anaesthetic drugs are vasodilators. However, before a patient is ready for discharge from the Recovery unit, the nursing and anaesthetic staff must satisfy themselves that these drugs have worn off. Opioids have relatively little effect on systemic vascular resistance, hence their liberal use in cardiac surgery, although they may cause mild or moderate hypotension in the elderly.

Central neuraxial blockade

Central neuraxial blockade includes spinal and epidural anaesthesia and analgesia. Epidural analgesia will be encountered on the ward most commonly after major abdominal surgery or orthopaedic or vascular surgery to the lower limb. A feature common to central neuraxial blockade is the sympathetic block due to blockade of outflow from the sympathetic chains in the thorax and abdomen, resulting in peripheral vasodilatation. It also follows that the higher the epidural block, the more extensive the sympathetic blockade, resulting in more hypotension.

Any patient with a working epidural in situ should have the dermatomal level of the block documented with an ice cube, as it may be much higher than necessary. If too high the rate of the infusion can be decreased. If this is not successful in improving hypotension then consider sympathomimetics, e.g. ephedrine in 3–6 mg boluses and fluids.

Remember:

1. Do not try to manage an epidural on your own, always enlist the help of an anaesthetist or pain nurse.

2. Hypotension may occur after a bolus dose of local anaesthetic injected into the epidural space. This may only become apparent after approximately 15 min.

3. Profound hypotension of rapid onset after a bolus injection of local anaesthetic in this setting may suggest inadvertant subarachnoid injection. Treatment of this again is sympathomimetics, fluids and other supportive measures.

4. Do not forget the prospect of local anaesthetic toxicity due to inadvertent intravascular injection of local anaesthetic. This may be seen especially with bupivacaine, which is notoriously cardiotoxic, causing cardiovascular collapse (see Chapter 18: Local anaesthetics).

However, in the presence of an epidural for postoperative pain control, the much more common causes of postoperative hypotension must not be ignored (e.g. bleeding and inadequate fluid resuscitation). An epidural is a poor excuse to allow prolonged postoperative hypotension – end organ damage can cause significant morbidity and mortality.

Sepsis

Sepsis should be considered in a setting of appropriate history, pyrexia, warm dilated peripheries, hypotension and extremes of white cell count. There may be associated cerebral and renal dysfunction characterised by confusion and renal impairment/failure. Treatment consists of identifying

25

the source, taking appropriate cultures and administering antibiotics and arranging other supportive therapy and specialist monitoring.

Adverse drug reactions and anaphylaxis

This may be evident from the history, e.g. the timing of hypotension relative to drug administration, e.g. antibiotics. The main treatment for anaphylaxis is to stop the drug administration immediately, give adrenaline (epinephrine) 1 mcg per kilogram intravenously with fluids and other supportive measures.

Key points

1. Postoperative hypotension is common.

2. Hypotension may be due to a variety of causes – do not immediately blame the epidural, it is far more likely to be hypovolaemia!

3. Prompt diagnosis and treatment are essential to prevent serious sequelae (e.g. myocardial ischaemia, oliguria).

4. Patients with postoperative epidural infusions need particular care during management of hypotension – involve the anaesthetist or pain nurse.

25

26

Postoperative complications

Dan Wheeler and Jeremy Lermitte

Complications can occur as part of any surgical admission. They can be distressing and inconvenient or life threatening. They are most likely to occur after major surgery or in patients with significant cardiac, respiratory, hepatic or renal morbidity. Complications causing single organ or system failure can lead inexorably to multiple system failure or even death. When resources and beds are scarce, treatment of complications occupies medical and nursing time, and increases length of hospital stay. They can also result in litigation.

Complications occur when organs begin to fail. Organs fail when:

■ they are not adequately perfused with blood

■ they are not supplied with sufficiently oxygenated blood

■ their function is diminished by toxins

■ they are affected by combinations of the above

Surgery injures and kills cells, causing inflammatory mediators like cytokines, thromboxanes, leukotrienes, prostaglandins, and nitric oxide to be released. This inflammatory response prevents introduction of infection into the body and promotes healing. An uncomplicated recovery from surgery relies on the body being able to increase its metabolic rate enough to maintain its normal homeostatic mechanisms and mount an adequate inflammatory response. A cell's normal source of energy is derived from adenosine triphosphate (ATP), created during the metabolism of glucose in the presence of oxygen.

26

Aerobic respiration	Anaerobic respiration
Requires presence of oxygen	Occurs when oxygen is absent or scarce
Requires presence of glucose	Requires presence of glucose
Begins with glycolysis: ■ Produces 2 ATP ■ End product is pyruvate	Begins with glycolysis: ■ Produces 2 ATP ■ End product is pyruvate
Pyruvate is converted into acetyl CoA in the presence of oxygen	Pyruvate is not converted to acetyl CoA as the process is dependent on the presence of oxygen
Acetyl CoA enters the tricarboxylic acid cycle, yielding a further 36 moles of ATP per mole of glucose	Pyruvate is converted to lactate
Final energy yield per mole of glucose	
38 moles ATP	2 moles ATP plus lactate

If oxygen or glucose is in short supply during or after surgery, cells will soon switch to anaerobic metabolism, producing so little ATP that membrane pumps fail. They swell and are eventually irreversibly damaged or ruptured. Those with high oxygen demand like myocardial cells, renal cells and neurons are especially susceptible. Most postoperative complications develop when organs fail to function correctly as oxygen supply to their cells does not meet demand.

The impact of complications can be reduced by identifying patients at risk, preoperative optimisation, appropriate postoperative monitoring and prompt treatment. On a physiological level, this can be thought of as providing cells with sufficient oxygen and glucose to meet their energy demands. This occurs when blood is adequately oxygenated and the heart can produce enough systolic pressure to perfuse the tissues. Clinically, patients must be assessed preoperatively to identify those at increased risk of postoperative hypoxaemia or organ hypoperfusion, so that their condition can be optimised and appropriate postoperative monitoring instituted (e.g. High Dependency Unit admission). Prompt identification of postoperative hypoxaemia or organ hypoperfusion and appropriate intervention limits the severity of complications and prevents the downward spiral into multi-organ failure.

This chapter discusses the physiological and pathophysiological basis of postoperative complications by reference to body systems. Several recurring themes throughout this book should be borne in mind at the same time: prevention of complications is better than cure; comprehensive preoperative assessment helps guide the choice of appropriate postoperative monitoring; and observations should be considered in the context of that patient's normal results and as part of a trend.

26

Cardiovascular physiology and cardiovascular complications

To avoid myocardial ischaemia the coronary arteries must be perfused with oxygenated blood at an adequate pressure. Most coronary blood flow, especially to the left ventricle, occurs in diastole but coronary perfusion is not solely determined by diastolic blood pressure. The coronary arteries are compressed from outside by pressure exerted by the blood that remains in the left ventricle in diastole. Outflow from the coronary arteries via the coronary sinus into the right atrium is diminished by high right-sided venous pressure. Therefore:

Coronary perfusion = diastolic arterial blood pressure
pressure   − left ventricular end diastolic pressure (LVEDP)
               − central venous pressure (CVP)

So coronary perfusion pressure is:

Increased by	Reduced by
Increasing (diastolic) blood pressure ■ arteriolar vasoconstriction	Reduced (diastolic) blood pressure ■ peripheral vasodilatation, e.g. sepsis, epidural block
Reducing LVEDP ■ improved cardiac output ■ increased myocardial contractility ■ increased ejection fraction ■ positive inotropic drugs	Increased LVEDP ■ cardiac failure ■ decreased myocardial contractility ■ decreased ejection fraction
Reducing CVP ■ venodilators	Increased CVP ■ cardiac failure

Another consideration is the amount of time available for coronary perfusion. Most coronary blood flow occurs in diastole. The length of systole is relatively fixed. When heart rate rises, diastole shortens and hence diastolic blood flow is reduced. A heart rate of $90\,min^{-1}$ is thought to provide optimal coronary blood flow.

The myocardium relies entirely on aerobic respiration and has a high oxygen demand. Another strategy is to decrease the myocardium's oxygen demand using β-blockers. There is increasing evidence that perioperative β-blockade reduces myocardial ischaemia in those with ischaemic heart disease. Hypertension and positive inotropic drugs increase myocardial work and therefore increase oxygen demand.

Blood pressure or blood flow?

To understand how the heart and other vital organs ensure their oxygen supply is maintained in the face of changing physiology, it is important to understand the relationship between blood pressure and blood flow. The healthy heart, kidneys, and brain are able to regulate their own blood flow at a local level. Autoregulation may occur as a result of:

■ *Myogenic factors* – smooth muscle in the arteriolar wall responds to changing intraluminal pressure by relaxing or contracting in such a way so as to maintain a constant radius and thus blood flow.

■ *Metabolic factors* – when blood flow is low, vasodilating factors such as nitric oxide, CO_2, adenosine and H^+ accumulate, causing vasodilatation and therefore increased blood flow.

■ *Tissue factors* – when blood flow is high, interstitial fluid accumulates in the vessel walls, which swell and reduce the diameter of the lumen.

26

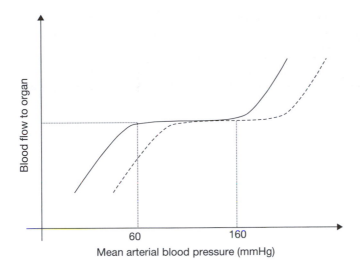

Mean arterial blood pressure (mmHg)

Blood flow is maintained across a wide range of arterial pressures. Chronic hypertension shifts the above curve to the right (dashed line), so relative hypotension can lead to decreased blood flow when a patient's blood pressure lies within the 'normal range'. In sepsis, critical illness or poststenotic dilatation, autoregulation can be lost, and the relationship between flow and pressure becomes linear. Under these circumstances a small fall in blood pressure can lead to a large fall in blood flow.

Therefore it is possible for a patient to have an acceptable blood pressure but poor blood flow, or a poor blood pressure but good blood flow. This is complicated by the fact that different regions of the circulation react in different ways to physiological changes, for example in shock the circulation to vital organs such as brain and heart are preserved and there is vasoconstriction in splanchnic and skeletal muscle vascular beds.

This is all very well but unfortunately it is very difficult to measure blood flow, especially to individual organs. Measuring systemic blood pressure is relatively simple but calculating organ perfusion pressures (coronary or cerebral) involves highly specialised invasive monitoring. The only way forward when managing ill patients is to:

- remember that a result or observation that lies within the 'normal range' might not represent normality

- adequate pressures may not represent adequate flows

- poor organ perfusion may only be detected by the onset of more subtle signs, symptoms or metabolic derangements than can be detected by routine bedside observations

- trust your or your nursing colleagues' intuition – if a patient looks ill, they probably are ill

26

More details about the recognition and management of the critically ill patient can be found in Chapter 14: The critically ill patient.

Myocardial ischaemia and infarction

Myocardial ischaemia occurs when *oxygen demand* is not met by *oxygen supply* and may lead to myocardial infarction. Using the framework above, the causative factors can be identified as:

■ hypoxaemia

■ arterial hypotension

■ cardiac failure

■ hypertension

■ tachycardia

The Goldman index of cardiac risk (see Chapter 1: Perioperative management of cardiovascular disease) identifies high-risk patients preoperatively, recognising cardiac failure, atrial dysrhythmias and myocardial infarction within the past 6 months as the greatest risk factors. Appropriate monitoring and the availability of a baseline preoperative ECG for comparison are essential because ischaemia or infarction may be asymptomatic. High-risk patients should have continuous ECG monitoring, daily 12-lead ECGs and serial measurement of cardiac injury markers.

T-wave inversion, ST segment changes or new bundle branch block on a 12-lead ECG indicate myocardial ischaemia or infarction. Postoperative myocardial infarction carries a mortality of 50%. The postoperative rise in creatine kinase resulting from surgery may mask myocardial injury; measurement of the MB isoenzyme fraction and troponin I levels are helpful in such circumstances. Treatment requires specialist help, especially if cardiogenic shock is present. Initial therapy should include 100% oxygen and analgesia. Thrombolysis is often contraindicated in the immediate postoperative period, but aspirin, β-blockers and heparinisation might be appropriate.

Ventricular failure

Starling described how a healthy heart optimises cardiac output by increasing myocardial contractility when venous return increases, in other words it matches preload with afterload. If the myocardium is ischaemic or diseased, or fluid overload increases preload precipitously, one or both ventricles can fail and cardiac output is embarrassed.

Tachycardia, tachypnoea, cyanosis, pulmonary oedema and even hypotension may be evident. Signs of right ventricular failure (e.g. raised jugular venous pressure, hepatomegaly) are seen in congestive or biventricular cardiac failure.

26

Reducing preload by decreasing venous return interrupts this vicious cycle. Basic principles of treatment include administration of supplemental oxygen at high concentration, and optimisation of preload and afterload with diuretics, opioids and nitrates. Elderly or severely ill patients may benefit from invasive haemodynamic monitoring, inotropes, and (in some cases) ventilatory support.

Rarely, only the right ventricle fails. This may be the consequence of a true posterior infarction (which involves the right ventricle) or pulmonary hypertension, which can be primary or secondary to the acute respiratory distress syndrome.

Cardiogenic shock

Occasionally the failing heart cannot maintain sufficient cardiac output to perfuse vital organs, despite normovolaemia and the absence of mechanical circulatory obstruction. This is termed as cardiogenic shock and has a mortality of 90%. Intensive care, invasive pressure monitoring, inotropes and ventilatory support may be beneficial.

Hypotension

Hypotension exists when blood pressure is too low to perfuse vital organs. If a patient's normal blood pressure is 190/100, 120/80 may represent hypotension. Symptoms of mild hypotension are nausea, vomiting and dizziness, and as it worsens there may be anxiety, confusion or even coma.

Postoperative hypotension can be caused by:

- hypovolaemia
- cardiac failure
- arrhythmias
- drugs
- spinal or epidural anaesthesia

26

The signs and treatment of each vary, but the sequelae are the same: persistent hypoperfusion of vital organs causes irreversible kidney, brain or gut failure. Hypotension is discussed in more detail in Chapter 25: Postoperative hypotension.

Arrhythmias

Supraventricular and ventricular arrhythmias are common during surgery, because general anaesthetics sensitise the myocardium to the effects of circulating catecholamines. Most are benign and self-limiting, but the aetiology of persistent or compromising arrhythmias should be established (Table 26.1).

Tachycardia increases myocardial oxygen demand and compromises left ventricular blood supply by reducing diastolic coronary artery filling time. Loss of coordinated atrial contraction reduces cardiac output by 20% and

Table 26.1 Causes of perioperative arrhythmias

Physiological disturbance
- Acidosis
- Hypercapnoea
- Hypoxaemia
- Electrolyte imbalance (especially K^+, Mg^{2+} abnormalities)
- Vagal manoeuvres
- Hypovolaemia

Pathological disturbance
- Pain
- Myocardial ischaemia or infarction
- Pulmonary embolus
- Phaeochromocytoma

Pharmacological causes
- General anaesthetics (sensitise myocardium to circulating catecholamines)
- Local anaesthetic toxicity
- Positive and negative inotropes

26

increases the risk of thromboembolism. Bradycardias and ventricular ectopics may compromise cardiac output.

Supplemental oxygen should be administered, blood pressure measured, diagnosis confirmed with a 12-lead ECG and rhythm strip, and help sought. The principles behind treatment algorithms are summarised in Table 26.2.

Conduction defects

General anaesthetics, electrolyte imbalances and local anaesthetic toxicity decrease atrioventricular nodal conduction perioperatively. Patients with certain heart blocks may thus develop complete heart block, compromising cardiac output. These must be identified on the preoperative ECG so that a temporary transvenous pacing wire can be inserted to treat complete heart block if it develops. For more detail see Chapter 1: Perioperative management of cardiovascular disease.

Drugs

The effects of residual general anaesthetic drugs in the postoperative period can decrease systemic vascular resistance or reduce cardiac output by directly depressing myocardial contractility. These effects do not usually

Table 26.2 Principles behind the management of postoperative arrhythmias

Basic action
- Administration of supplemental oxygen
- Pulse present?
- Blood pressure compromised?

Diagnosis
- 12-lead ECG and rhythm strip
- Tachycardia or bradycardia?
- Supraventricular or ventricular?

Urgency of treatment
- Cardiopulmonary resuscitation needed?
- Help needed?
- Time to treat easily reversible cause?

Cardioversion
- DC cardioversion
- Cardioversion with drugs
- Rate control

persist beyond the immediate postoperative period, and are seldom important once the patient has left the recovery area.

Epidural and spinal local anaesthetic blocks sympathetic nerves to blood vessels, and cause persistent vasodilatation and hypotension that may persist after the patient returns to the ward, especially if the regional block is used to provide postoperative analgesia. The patient may be slightly tachycardic, with warm, well-perfused peripheries. A fluid challenge and elevation of the legs should restore blood pressure, but the level of the epidural block and adequacy of analgesia should be checked.

Hypertension

Postoperative hypertension can be caused by:

- pain
- pre-existing essential hypertension, especially if poorly controlled
- hypoxaemia
- hypercapnoea
- iatrogenic over-administration of positive inotropes

26

221

Hypertension increases afterload, increasing myocardial work and oxygen demand. Hence, it can precipitate myocardial ischaemia or infarction. It may also lead to stroke. After optimisation of analgesia, the blood pressure should be reassessed in the context of that documented preoperatively. Oxygen should be administered, and blood pressure in chronically hypertensive patients controlled with their usual therapy or a substitute if it cannot be tolerated or delivered. Occasionally, hypertension may present for the first time in the perioperative period, and require specific therapy. The anti-hypertensive chosen depends on each scenario and which class of drug is tolerated best. Treating hypertension can unmask hypovolaemia and some patients may require more fluids.

Respiratory system

Postoperative changes in a patient's ventilation, lung volumes, gas exchange and immune defences can lead to complications.

Ventilation

Hypoventilation leads to hypoxaemia and hypercapnoea. It can be caused by airway obstruction, decreased ventilatory drive, pain, or weakness of the peripheral respiratory muscles. Residual general anaesthetic, opioids and inadequately reversed neuromuscular blockade blunt the response to hypercapnoea. Patients should not be discharged from the recovery area until they can maintain a safe airway and a normal respiratory pattern.

Opioids cause hypoventilation by depressing central respiratory drive. Patients who have received long-acting intrathecal opioids (e.g. spinal diamorphine), those on opioid infusions, or those with concurrent conditions (e.g. obesity, intracranial pathology) are most at risk. Opioid delivery by patient-controlled analgesia systems (PCA) is safer but can still cause hypoventilation or airway obstruction. Most hospitals have specific protocols to detect hypoventilation in patients on PCA. Such protocols trigger emergency anaesthetic referral and/or administration of the opioid receptor antagonist, naloxone.

Lung volumes

During and after thoracic and major abdominal surgery the vital capacity is reduced by 45% and functional residual capacity by 20% as a result of diaphragmatic splinting and wound pain. These changes cause alveolar collapse, atelectasis and shunting, all of which are more pronounced in the elderly or obese. Right to left shunt due to alveolar collapse should be treated with supplemental oxygen but strategies to re-expand collapsed areas are also required. These may include physiotherapy, optimising analgesia and continuous positive airway pressure (CPAP).

26

Table 26.3 Causes of postoperative impairment of gas exchange

Lack of alveolar ventilation
- Hypoventilation (airway obstruction, opioids)

- Bronchospasm

- Pneumothorax

- Shunting (alveolar collapse, atelectasis)

Lack of alveolar perfusion
- Ventilation-perfusion mismatch (pulmonary embolism)

- Impaired cardiac output

Decreased diffusion across alveolar membrane
- Pneumonia

- Pulmonary oedema

- Acute respiratory distress syndrome (ARDS) and inflammation

Gas exchange
Impaired gas exchange across the alveolar membrane, ventilation-perfusion mismatching or lack of alveolar ventilation also cause hypercapnoea and hypoxaemia (Table 26.3)

Impaired immune defences
Several factors combine to cause respiratory mucosal damage perioperatively, increasing risk of infection. Breathing non-humidified oxygen dries protective secretions; drugs and pain impair the cough reflex. General anaesthetics suppress the mucociliary escalator and impair granulocyte function *in vitro*. High inflation pressures during ventilation exacerbate damage.

Pneumonia
Patients recovering from major surgery may acquire nosocomial bronchopneumonia owing to impaired immune defence or prolonged ventilation. Lobar pneumonia is uncommon, but can be caused by aspiration when the airway is not secured in obtunded patients. Causative organisms are often atypical, including *Pseudomonas aeruginosa* and anaerobes, and are difficult to treat.

Pulmonary embolus
When peripheral venous thromboses embolise to the pulmonary artery, symptoms and signs vary widely (Table 26.4). The easiest investigations to perform are the least specific. ECG may show the classical '$S_IQ_{III}T_{III}$' right ventricular strain pattern or just sinus tachycardia. Arterial blood gases

26

Table 26.4 Symptoms and signs of pulmonary embolus

	Occurrence (%)
Symptoms	
■ Dyspnoea	77
■ Chest pain	63
■ Haemoptysis	26
■ Classic triad of all three symptoms	14
Signs	
■ Tachycardia	59
■ Fever	43
■ Tachypnoea	38
■ Signs of deep venous thrombosis	23
■ Raised jugulovenous pressure	18
■ Shock	11
■ Accentuated second pulmonary heart sound	11
■ Cyanosis	9
■ Pleural friction rub	8

26

may document ventilation-perfusion mismatching by showing hypoxaemia in the presence of *hypocapnoea*, but are often normal. Chest radiographs seldom show oligaemic lung fields. Ventilation-perfusion scanning can be diagnostic, but atelectasis and pneumonia can make interpretation difficult. Conventional pulmonary angiography is the gold standard for diagnosis, but is not widely available. Spiral CT with contrast can provide excellent pulmonary angiograms, and is increasingly being seen as a definitive diagnostic tool in pulmonary embolus. Anti-coagulation with heparin followed by warfarin is the mainstay of treatment. Rarely, thrombolysis or embolectomy may be required.

Pneumothorax
An attempt at central venous access or brachial plexus block can result in pneumothorax, which should be excluded by a chest radiograph. Pneumothorax can also be caused by barotrauma when high airway pressures are required to artificially ventilate non-compliant lungs, for example in bronchospasm, chronic obstructive pulmonary disease (COPD), ARDS, pulmonary oedema or as a result of medical error.

Monitoring and treatment of postoperative respiratory failure

Patients identified as being at high risk of hypoxaemia postoperatively should have peripheral oxygen saturation monitored continuously. An oxygen saturation of less than 92% *while on supplemental oxygen* is a cause for concern and should trigger the measurement of arterial blood gases, *without removing the supplemental oxygen*. Interpretation of arterial blood gases is covered in Chapter 16: Arterial blood gases.

Any cause of hypoxaemia should be treated with supplemental oxygen delivered continuously by fixed-performance mask. Other masks and nasal prongs deliver varying concentrations of oxygen, dependent on peak inspiratory flow. Ventilation may be required if hypoxaemia does not respond to high oxygen concentrations, or if the patient is tiring.

A minority of patients with COPD retain CO_2, and can be rendered apnoeic by high oxygen concentrations. Most patients with chronic lung disease are undertreated with oxygen for this reason. Regular measurement of arterial blood gases allows the detection of the onset of hypercapnoea under these circumstances. Management in such patients is facilitated by the measurement of arterial gases in the preoperative period, providing a baseline reference value for comparison.

The central nervous system

The physiological principles determining blood flow and oxygen delivery to the brain are similar to that of the heart. The brain has the ability to autoregulate its blood flow, and has very high oxygen consumption. The brain, cerebral blood vessels and cerebrospinal fluid (CSF) are contained in a rigid box (the cranium), which has important implications for cerebral blood flow. Brain tissue and CSF exert pressure on the cerebral blood vessels from without, so that:

26

Cerebral perfusion pressure = mean arterial blood pressure
− intracranial pressure (ICP)
− central venous pressure (CVP)

So cerebral perfusion pressure is:

Increased by	Reduced by
Increasing arterial blood pressure	Reducing arterial blood pressure
Reducing ICP ■ hyperventilation ■ CSF drains	Increasing ICP ■ hypercapnoea ■ hypoxia ■ coughing, straining, fitting ■ space occupying lesion

Increased by	Reduced by
Reducing CVP	Increasing CVP ■ cardiac failure ■ obstruction to jugular venous drainage, e.g. raised intrathoracic pressure, tight endotracheal tube ties

Like the heart, the brain relies entirely on aerobic respiration and has a high oxygen demand. However, reducing cerebral oxygen demand is not so straightforward. Most drugs used to achieve this are sedatives, anaesthetic agents or anti-convulsants, which depress breathing so much that the patient requires artificial ventilation on intensive care.

The brain is also susceptible to the detrimental effects of toxins, electrolyte and metabolic disturbances.

'Brain failure'

Heart failure is a term used frequently and is well understood. 'Brain failure' may be manifest as:

■ coma and unconsciousness

■ confusion and agitation

■ cerebrovascular accident (infarction or intracerebral haemorrhage)

■ convulsions

It occurs due to imbalance of oxygen demand and supply or the presence of specific toxins.

Coma and unconsciousness

In the recovery area, the metabolism and elimination of anaesthetic drugs should result in a progressive improvement in conscious state until the patient is alert and orientated. Recovery from anaesthesia may be delayed if drugs with long half-lives, benzodiazepines or barbiturates have been administered. Even in such cases, however, the trend is for the conscious level to improve, and any deterioration in conscious state should trigger further action, rather than attributing the clinical picture to residual anaesthetic effects. If a patient becomes unresponsive postoperatively, immediate action is required to maintain a safe airway and ensure adequate breathing and circulation. Table 26.5 summarises the possible causes.

Confusion and agitation

The elderly are particularly prone to postoperative confusion, and almost any diagnosis can present in this way. Many of the causes of coma can also account for confusion. Hypoxaemia, pain and electrolyte imbalance are the most common causes and are easily treated. In addition, the elderly are

26

Table 26.5 Causes of postoperative unconsciousness

Hypoxaemia
- Cerebral ischaemia
- Coma resulting from hypoxaemia is a preterminal sign

Hypercapnoea
- Arterial CO_2 tensions of $>9\,kPa$ lead to coma

Hypotension
- Hypoperfusion exacerbates cerebral ischaemia

Cerebrovascular accident
- Intracranial haemorrhage
- Thrombo-embolic infarction
- Raised intracranial pressure in the presence of head injury, tumour

Endocrine
- Hypoglycaemia
- Hyperglycaemia
- Hypothyroidism
- Addisonian crisis

Hypo-osmolar syndrome
- Hyponatraemia resulting from absorption of water during bladder or rectal irrigation with glycine-containing fluids

Drugs
- Residual anaesthetic drugs
- Opioid analgesics
- Benzodiazepines
- Intracranial spread of local anaesthetic from epidural or interscalene block

Toxins
- Alcohol
- Illicit drugs
- Ammonia (hepatic encephalopathy, renal failure)

Air embolus
- Neurosurgical patients at high risk

Epilepsy
- Post ictal

Hypothermia
- Profound hypothermia causes coma

26

prone to confusion secondary to toxins and drugs. Alcohol and benzodiazepine withdrawal should be considered along with a central anti-cholinergic syndrome caused by lipid-soluble drugs (e.g. atropine, cyclizine).

Cerebrovascular accident

When oxygen delivery to the brain is insufficient to meet cerebral oxygen demand, neurons eventually become irreparably damaged. Any cause of profound hypoxaemia or hypotension can cause global or focal brain injury. Thrombo-embolic or haemorrhagic stroke may occur perioperatively, especially in patients with hypertension, atrial arrhythmia or arteriosclerosis.

Headache

Mild headache is an inconvenient complication of general anaesthesia. Dural puncture and CSF leakage during spinal or epidural anaesthesia can cause severe intractable headache. Its distribution is occipital and frontal and it is exacerbated by bright lights, and sitting or bending forwards. Post dural puncture headache can occur weeks after surgery and persist for months. Treatment includes rest, hydration and simple analgesics. Failure of initial treatment may indicate the need for an epidural blood patch.

Peripheral nervous system

Prolonged neuromuscular block

26

Suxamethonium is a depolarising neuromuscular blocking drug, widely used in rapid sequence induction of anaesthesia. It is metabolised by plasma cholinesterase and its half-life is 3 minutes, but the plasma levels of the enzyme may be reduced in some patients owing to autosomally inherited genetic defects. In extreme examples, homozygotes remain paralysed for many hours and require sedation and ventilation.

Peripheral nerve palsies

Careful patient positioning is paramount to avoid nerve palsies. Pressure at the elbow can cause ulnar nerve neuropraxia, and incorrect lithotomy positioning can cause obturator, femoral or common peroneal nerve neuropraxia. Spinal and epidural anaesthesia seldom result in neural injury, and nerve injury from peripheral nerve blocks is uncommon. Using stimulator needles for peripheral blocks and performing epidurals or spinals when patients are awake and thus alert the onset of paraesthesia helps to minimise the incidence of these complications.

Rare neurological complications of epidurals and spinals

Instrumentation of the epidural space can damage the epidural venous plexus. Very rarely a haematoma may form, compressing the spinal cord or cauda equina. Severe pain and pressure at the epidural site, urinary retention and distal lower motor neurone deficit may be masked by subsequent epidural infusion of local anaesthetic. CT or MRI is diagnostic. The haematoma requires emergency evacuation to prevent permanent damage. Epidurals and spinals are contraindicated in coagulopathy, thrombocytopenia and full anti-coagulation. Prophylactic heparin should be withheld for at least 8 hours before regional anaesthesia.

Epidural abscess is rare but serious, developing days or weeks after epidural or spinal anaesthesia. Symptoms are similar, but examination may reveal an inflamed, hot, tender or discharging epidural site. Imaging, followed by surgical evacuation and/or antibiotics are the mainstays of treatment. Permanent neurological damage can also be caused by the development of meningitis, transverse myelitis or cauda equina syndrome.

Gastrointestinal system

Hepatic dysfunction

Halothane-induced hepatic necrosis is rare, but is associated with a mortality of 40%. Patients exhibit signs of hepatocellular jaundice with elevated serum aminotransferases. The damage may be related to the high proportion of halothane metabolised by the liver. Newer anaesthetic agents (e.g. isoflurane) are metabolised less and have a much lower risk of causing hepatitis. Table 26.6 shows the more common causes of postoperative hepatic dysfunction.

26

Table 26.6 **Causes of postoperative hepatic dysfunction**

Increased bilirubin load
- Blood transfusion
- Haemolysis
- Haemolytic disease
- Abnormalities of bilirubin metabolism

Hepatocellular damage
- Pre-existing hepatic disease
- Viral hepatitis
- Sepsis
- Hypotension
- Hypoxaemia
- Drug-induced hepatitis

Table 26.6 (continued)

■ Congestive cardiac failure

■ Hepatic necrosis secondary to general anaesthetics

Extrahepatic biliary obstruction
■ Gallstones

■ Ascending cholangitis

■ Pancreatitis

■ Common bile duct injury

Genitourinary system

Renal failure

Patients with existing renal impairment, renovascular disease, diabetes mellitus, sepsis or hypotension are most at risk of developing renal failure perioperatively.

The physiological model applied to perfusion and oxygenation of the heart and brain also applies to the kidneys. They:

■ can autoregulate their blood supply

■ have a high oxygen demand

■ can be affected by toxins

■ are subject to macroscopic and microscopic influences on their perfusion

Renal perfusion pressure = mean arterial blood pressure
− intra-abdominal pressure − CVP

Filtration in the glomerulus depends on:

■ glomerular surface area – vasoconstrictors (noradrenaline, vasopressin, angiotensin II, prostaglandins, leukotrienes) reduce the area available for filtration

■ permeability of the glomerulus – normally small molecules ≤6–8 nm pass freely from blood to filtrate, but if there is disease of the basement membrane or podocytes larger molecules may be lost from the blood, e.g. albumin in nephrotic syndrome

■ hydrostatic pressure gradient across the glomerulus – determined by renal blood flow and the difference between afferent arteriolar tone and efferent arteriolar tone

■ obstruction to urinary outflow, e.g. ureteric or urethral obstruction

26

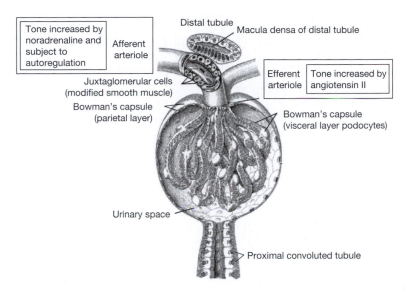

Tone increased by noradrenaline and subject to autoregulation

Afferent arteriole

Distal tubule

Macula densa of distal tubule

Efferent arteriole | Tone increased by angiotensin II

Juxtaglomerular cells (modified smooth muscle)

Bowman's capsule (parietal layer)

Bowman's capsule (visceral layer podocytes)

Urinary space

Proximal convoluted tubule

From Junqueira LC, Carneiro J and Kelley RO. Basic Histology, 8th ed. Appleton & Lange, 1996.

A rising creatinine perioperatively therefore indicates acute renal impairment, and that the pathology may be:

Prerenal failure (hypoperfusion)

■ Hypotension or shock (hypovolaemia, cardiogenic, septic)

■ Renal artery disease or obstruction

Renal (direct injury)

■ Glomerular:

- glomerulonephritis

- diabetes mellitus

- amyloidosis

■ Tubulointerstitial:

- acute tubular necrosis (follows prerenal failure, aminoglycosides, contrast medium, myoglobin)

- acute cortical necrosis (pre-eclampsia, septic abortion, placental abruption)

- interstitial nephritis (antibiotics)

■ Vascular:

- connective tissue disease

- hypertension

26

Postrenal failure (obstruction)

■ Bladder outflow (enlarged prostate, urethral stricture)

■ Single ureter (calculus, tumour, papilla, iatrogenic)

■ Both ureters (bladder malignancy)

> Renal failure = renal impairment + symptoms

Symptoms of renal failure

■ Nausea and vomiting

■ Malaise

■ Increased bleeding

■ Uraemic encephalopathy

■ Poor wound healing

■ Susceptibility to infection

Signs of renal failure

■ Oliguria (urine output = <1 ml/kg/h in infants, <0.5 ml/kg/h in children and <400 ml/day in adults)

■ Oedema

■ Hypertension

■ Acidosis

■ Hyperkalaemia

Urine output greater than or equal to 1 ml/kg/h is considered adequate. Renal failure can develop despite adequate urine output, so serum urea and creatinine should be measured regularly in patients at risk.

Rising urea and creatinine levels and/or a falling urine output that is not artefactual (e.g. a blocked catheter) or extrarenal in origin (urea elevation owing to a gastrointestinal bleed) should prompt further investigation and therapy.

Examination of the urine may help differentiate between different causes of renal failure:

■ Microscopy: tubular casts visible in acute tubular necrosis

■ Measurement of urinary myoglobin levels

The following test the concentrating ability of the kidneys. If the kidneys are able to concentrate they will excrete urine with high osmolality and specific gravity, low urinary sodium (high aldosterone levels stimulate water reabsorption via retention of Na^+ in the distal tubule), and high concentrations of urea and creatinine when compared to plasma. These findings are compatible with prerenal failure.

26

In renal failure, concentrating ability is lost. Urine is dilute, high in sodium and contains urea and creatinine levels closer to that of plasma.

Investigation	Prerenal failure	Renal failure
Urinary specific gravity	>1.020	<1.010
Urine osmolality (mosmol/kg)	>500	<350
Urine sodium (mmol/l)	<20	>40
Urine/plasma osmolality ratio	>2	<1.1
Urine/plasma urea ratio	>20	<10
Urine/plasma creatinine ratio	>40	<20

The frameworks given above also guide treatment:

■ monitor urine output (hourly), weight (daily), urea and creatinine, acid-base status

■ renal perfusion should be optimised with volume replacement, haemodynamic monitoring and inotropes where appropriate

■ to prevent fluid overload a reasonable replacement strategy is to restrict intravenous fluid replacement to the previous hour's urine output plus 25–30 ml to account for insensible losses.

■ urinary obstruction should be excluded

■ nephrotoxic drugs should be discontinued

26

Frusemide, which decreases renal cell oxygen demand, and mannitol, which scavenges damaging free radicals, are often administered to protect the kidneys. Dopamine is thought to improve renal blood flow by dilating the renal vascular bed. Although there is no doubt that these drugs increase urine output, there is little evidence that they can avert decline into renal failure or improve outcome.

Renal replacement therapy

Renal replacement therapy may be necessary if hyperkalaemia, circulating volume, or symptoms of renal failure cannot be controlled.

Dialysis is the removal of solutes and water from the blood using a semipermeable membrane across which solutes move according to osmotic or hydrostatic gradients, and can be manipulated by altering those gradients. Dialysis may be:

■ *Peritoneal* – A hypertonic solution is introduced into the peritoneum via an indwelling catheter and allowed to equilibrate with plasma and is then drained away, exploiting the peritoneum as the semipermeable membrane. It is simple, does not require vascular access or anti-coagulation but is slow and less efficient than other techniques.

■ *Haemodialysis* – Blood passes through an extracorporeal circuit to a cellophane or fibrous membrane. The dialysate passes on the other side of the membrane in a counter-current system. Solutes are removed by diffusion into the dialysate, water is removed by application of a pressure gradient across the membrane (ultrafiltration). Requires vascular access via indwelling intravascular catheters or an arteriovenous shunt, and anti-coagulation. There can be problems with air bubbles or clots in the circuit, hypotension, and electrolyte and acid-base disturbance.

■ *Haemofiltration* – Blood is pumped via an extracorporeal circuit through a polyamide filter with a high surface area. A hydrostatic pressure gradient across the filter leads to ultrafiltration and drainage of water to the waste side of the filter; solutes follow down concentration gradients. The requirements for haemofiltration are much the same as haemodialysis, and many of the complications are shared, but haemofiltration does not cause such cardiovascular instability. Its efficiency can be further improved by passing dialysate through the waste side of the filter (haemodiafiltration). In haemoperfusion, waste molecules are adsorbed onto an ion exchange resin or activated charcoal. This also allows lipid soluble waste products to be removed.

26

Musculoskeletal system

Hypothermia
Patients in theatre lose heat to the atmosphere by convection, conduction, radiation and evaporation, and are further cooled by the administration of intravenous fluids at room temperature. Hypothermia decreases cardiac output, diminishes peripheral perfusion and deranges coagulation. Core temperature measurement and active patient and fluid warming are important in lengthy operations.

Shivering
Shivering in the postoperative period is commonly a compensatory response to the development of intraoperative hypothermia. Volatile general anaesthetics can result in postoperative shaking unrelated to hypothermia, and epidural anaesthesia may cause shivering. The muscular activity associated with shivering increases skeletal muscle oxygen utilisation and may cause hypoxaemia. Therapy includes oxygen supplementation and active warming to normothermia. Small doses of intravenous pethidine may be useful in intractable cases.

Malignant hyperpyrexia

General anaesthetics and suxamethonium trigger massive increases in metabolic rate in this rare heritable muscle disorder. Rhabdomyolysis and hyperpyrexia cause hypoxaemia, fits, hyperkalaemia and renal failure up to 8 hours after exposure. Prompt administration of dantrolene and 100% oxygen can reduce mortality from 70% to 20%.

Rhabdomyolysis

Rhabdomyolysis is the breakdown of muscle caused by:

- compartment syndrome

- crush injury

- prolonged ischaemia or immobility, e.g. aortic cross clamping, poisoning, overdose

- malignant hyperpyrexia

- hypothermia

- massive myocardial infarction

Myoglobin and creatine kinase are released. In acid urine, myoglobin breaks down into ferrihemate, which is nephrotoxic. Myoglobin is a small molecule that is freely filtered in the glomerulus but may aggregate in the renal tubules causing obstruction and acute tubular necrosis.

Rhabdomyolysis and myoglobinuria are usually diagnosed when a patient's urine is noted to be a deep red colour or serum creatine kinase is very elevated (in the tens of thousands). Biochemical testing of the urine confirms the presence of myoglobin. Treatment is to ensure a high urine output to prevent myoglobin aggregating, and administration of bicarbonate to alkalinise the urine to prevent the formation of ferrihemate. The need for close monitoring of acid-base status, renal function and hydration status demands admission to a High Dependency or Intensive Care Unit.

26

27

Perioperative scenarios

Dan Wheeler and Parameswaran Pillai

Seven 'grey' cases are presented to highlight important themes in the recognition and management of patients with perioperative complications or critical illness. The differential diagnoses are not exhaustive but aim to emphasise common problems encountered in clinical practice.

Advances in surgical and anaesthetic techniques mean that patients with significant co-morbidity are now undergoing elective surgery as a matter of routine when 10 or 20 years ago they would have been told that they were not fit for anaesthesia. Healthy patients are increasingly operated upon in Day Surgery. Nursing and medical staff on surgical wards are increasingly expected to recognise, treat and/or refer patients with a wide variety of co-morbid medical problems.

New working patterns mean that patients experience less continuity of care from medical staff. Junior doctors are increasingly likely to cross-cover other teams' patients whom they may never have met before, with problems that they have never seen before. Experienced nurses provide continuity and are much better at detecting the early signs of critical illness than doctors just starting out in their career. If a nurse asks a doctor to see and assess a patient, he or she should do so and not be tempted to dismiss their anxieties over the telephone just because the patient's observations lie within the 'normal range'. Finally, don't be afraid to ask for help.

1. You are a House Officer covering the surgical wards on a Sunday afternoon. Sister calls you to the ward to review a 69-year-old patient complaining of chest pain who underwent a hemicolectomy 3 days earlier.

What is your first action?
Ask Sister to kindly record another ECG and repeat the vital signs. If the patient has a history of ischaemic heart disease and there are no other contra-indications, prescribe sub-lingual GTN 0.5 mg over the telephone and start 100% oxygen.

What are you thinking on the way to the ward?
You start analysing the problem with the information you have. Old age, third postoperative day and hemicolectomy should arouse suspicion that the patient is developing one of several important postoperative complications associated with high morbidity and mortality. Causes include angina, myocardial infarction, pulmonary embolus, dissecting aortic aneurysm, pneumonia, pneumothorax, gastro-oesophageal reflux and costochondritis.

On the ward you find the patient to be an obese gentleman with a previous history of heavy smoking.

What are the salient points in the history that you will take?
You need to take a detailed history of the pain. When did it start, where is it, does it radiate, what is its nature, has he had similar pain before, are

there any relieving or exacerbating factors, is it associated with sweating, nausea, dizziness or dyspnoea? Take a past medical history to cover symptoms and signs of angina, myocardial infarction (MI), pulmonary embolus (PE), pneumothorax, pleurisy, pneumonia, oesophageal spasm, oesophagitis, gastritis, cholecystitis, costochondritis, etc. Remember to get all details about the medications that he is on which will give valuable clues. Look for any helpful clues in the medical or nursing notes or in the bedside charts.

The patient felt tightness across the chest while he tried to get out of bed. He had felt some chest pain nearly 2 years back, but never had such severe tightness before. He was advised to take some blood thinning tablets by his GP, but they did not agree with his ulcer, so he is on something else. Lying down relieved his pain and it felt like a tight band around the chest. He has developed a bad cough since operation and brings up phlegm.

What are you looking for on examination?

The examination should start with general examination and **then** proceed to specific system examination. Listen for pleural and pericardial rubs which are often missed. Consider pneumothorax especially if central venous access has been attempted, although this is less likely on the third postoperative day. A small pneumothorax might be difficult to detect clinically.

On examination the cardiovascular and respiratory systems are unremarkable.

Heart rate	90/min
Blood pressure	110/78 mmHg
JVP	not raised
Respiratory rate	12/min
Temperature	37.8°C

27

What investigations will you order and why?

Full blood count (FBC): looking for anaemia, which will reduce oxygen supply to the myocardium and neutrophilia that may point to infective pathology.

Urea and electrolytes (U&E): moderately raised urea and creatinine will suggest dehydration that contributes to reduce filling pressures of the heart.

Cardiac enzymes: difficult to interpret postoperatively, due to CK release from skeletal muscle. CK-MB fraction or troponin levels are more specific.

Arterial blood gases (ABG): to rule out hypoxia, hyper/hypocarbia, acidosis. These can increase the myocardial work and precipitate MI. Hypocarbia may point to PE. It is important to interpret ABGs with the F_iO_2 and the whole clinical picture in mind.

Electrocardiograph (ECG): always compare with a recent previous ECG. All patients of this age and undergoing this type of surgery should have had one done preoperatively. Specifically look for any new arrhythmias or conduction delays like left bundle branch block (LBBB).

Chest X-ray: this patient has all the predisposing factors to develop basal atelectasis and pneumonia: obesity, smoking, gastrointestinal surgery, and the fact that it is the immediate postoperative period. A chest X-ray will help to diagnose it and will also help to rule out pulmonary oedema.

His results are as follows:

Hb	9.8 g/dl
Hct	0.33
WBC	13.5×10^9/l
RBC	4.14×10^9/l
Platelets	198×10^9/l
plasma sodium	140 mmol/l
plasma potassium	3.8 mmol/l
plasma chloride	119 mmol/l
plasma urea	15.2 mmol/l
plasma creatinine	130 μmol/l
creatine kinase	310 IU/l
Arterial blood gases (ABGs), on 10 l/min O_2 via facemask:	
pH	7.30
pCO_2	5.23 kPa
P_aO_2	9.84 kPa
plasma bicarbonate	18.5 mmol/l
base excess	−5.3 mmol/l
S_aO_2	94.0%
ECG	New LBBB

27

Have any of the investigations helped you make a diagnosis?

The development of new LBBB on the ECG indicates that this patient has had an MI, probably precipitated by anaemia, dehydration, mild acidosis and an infective focus most probably in the lungs. CK-MB and troponin levels will confirm this. Postoperative myocardial ischaemia is often atypical or 'silent'. It may be masked by opioid analgesic drugs. Have a very low index of suspicion and record an ECG in all postoperative patients with chest pain, even if it seems to be eased by antacids or alginates. Research into the incidence of postoperative myocardial ischaemia is demonstrating that it is surprisingly common.

Who will you call for help?

Referral to the Medical Registrar as a matter of urgency, via your senior.

What is the basic management of this condition?

The basics should not be forgotten. For acute perioperative MI, sit the patient up and give them high concentration oxygen and opioid analgesia. Ask the Medical Registrar about aspirin. Thrombolysis is contra-indicated.

2. *As the surgical House Officer on night duty, you are asked to review an 84-year-old lady, as her urine output was 8 ml, 5 ml and nil for the last 3 h. She had a perforated duodenal ulcer (DU) operated upon this afternoon and the anaesthetist has specified to keep urine output >40 ml/h and give a unit of Gelofusine if output was <40 ml for two consecutive hours. She was on diclofenac for osteoarthritis of the knee and it is thought to have caused the DU. Her other problems include hypertension and mild angina and she is on atenolol for this.*

What are the possible causes?

This is a very common scenario encountered in postoperative patients. The challenge is to determine whether this is a prerenal or renal problem. The possible pathologies include dehydration, and/or hypotension leading to prerenal failure or exacerbation of NSAID-induced renal failure. Determining her intravascular volume status is of prime importance. Postrenal obstruction is unlikely in this case, but if a patient is anuric after a procedure during which the ureters or bladder may be damaged, for example major gynaecological, urological or bowel surgery, the presence or absence of hydronephrosis should be established by means of emergency abdominal ultrasound.

Does the history help you to decide her fluid status?

While assessing the fluid status of any patient, it is important to analyse the input and output. Fluid input will have been documented in the medical and/or nursing notes and anaesthetic chart. Determining the output and losses can be difficult. Presence of drains, fever, etc. may confuse the picture. In a patient who had a recent laparotomy, it is important to note how well fluid resuscitated she was before the operation! Elderly patients and those with cardiac history are frequently under filled postoperatively due to worries about cardiac failure.

What are you looking for on examination to confirm your suspicions?

This case illustrates how difficult it can be to assess a patient's fluid status by clinical means alone. But it is always useful to have a structured approach and make a diagnosis by gathering different pieces of evidence, each with their own particular pitfalls.

Heart rate: Usually tachycardia is expected. But beta-blockade and ischaemic heart disease may prevent a tachycardic response in this patient.

Blood pressure: It could be low, normal or raised. None of these give a definitive answer as to the patient's fluid status. Low blood pressure might

27

be due to dehydration or cardiogenic shock. Raised blood pressure can co-exist with dehydration or cardiac failure. The presence of a postural variation in blood pressure may be more significant, but on her first postoperative night this lady is unlikely to be able to get out of her bed.

Dry mouth, thirst: Patients in cardiac failure often feel thirsty. The mouth may be dry due to the anticholinergic effect of many of the anaesthetic or analgesic drugs used.

Skin turgor: Notoriously difficult to assess, especially in old age.

Pulmonary crepitations: These could be due to fluid overload, basal atelectasis, pneumonia or preexisting pulmonary fibrosis.

Ankle swelling: Patients in right heart failure and those who are fluid overloaded usually develop peripheral oedema. But other important factors determining the development of oedema are the balance between intravascular hydrostatic and oncotic pressures and the permeability of capillaries. Patients with peripheral oedema can still be intravascular volume depleted.

She has been complaining of dry mouth since she got back from recovery. Her skin is wrinkled but turgor cannot be appreciated. Auscultation of the chest reveals reduced air entry at bases bilaterally, with some crepitations. No rhonchi are heard. There is mild pitting oedema of both ankles and she confirms that her ankles were swollen even before the operation.

Heart rate	64/min
Blood pressure	110/74 mmHg
JVP	not raised

What investigations will you order and why?

There is no single investigation that will diagnose the fluid status of a patient. Again as with history we need to pick up clues from different investigations. Test results that appear within the normal range should be interpreted with caution and bearing in mind the different pathologies co-existing in our patient.

FBC: Hb and haematocrit are useful to differentiate between fluid overload and dehydration. But co-existing anaemia and dehydration will complicate the picture by producing normal results for both these tests.

U&E: Urea, creatinine and the ratio of the two will help to identify the picture. In dehydration urea will be disproportionately high compared to creatinine, although this is also seen in upper gastrointestinal haemorrhage due to reabsorption of haemoglobin in the small bowel.

Hb	11.0 g/dl
Hct	0.39
WBC	$11.5 \times 10^9/l$
Platelets	$235 \times 10^9/l$
plasma sodium	144 mmol/l
plasma potassium	4.8 mmol/l
plasma chloride	119 mmol/l
plasma urea	35.5 mmol/l
plasma creatinine	185 μmol/l

What would you do?

All the clinical signs and investigations suggest intravascular hypovolaemia resulting in prerenal failure, so this patient requires fluid replacement. In most patients, fluid administration can be guided by measuring hourly urine output. The ideal urine output in these circumstances is 1 ml/kg/h. Fluid management becomes difficult if patients have co-existing prerenal and renal parenchymal disease and you should ask for expert help. Such patients will not be able to produce an adequate urine output even if their intravascular volume depletion is corrected. They are at risk of being given too much fluid, which might precipitate cardiac failure in the elderly or those with ischaemic heart disease. This lady has a history of cardiac failure (ankle oedema) and might have sustained renal parenchymal damage as a result of old age and/or taking an NSAID.

It is ideal to have central venous pressure (CVP) monitoring to guide fluid therapy in these circumstances. CVP readings should be interpreted with caution. A single reading is of no real value. CVP readings are used mainly to look at a trend and to assess the response to an intervention. Even if this patient's first CVP reading lies within the 'normal' range (5–10 cmH$_2$O, 4–7 mmHg), a fluid challenge is warranted. Further fluid management will depend on the response to fluid challenge.

Usually three scenarios emerge from a fluid challenge (250 ml of a crystalloid infused over 10 min)

a. CVP does not rise or the rise is about 2 cmH$_2$O and is not sustained for 15 min. This indicates intravascular hypovolaemia.

b. CVP rises by 2–5 cmH$_2$O and the rise is sustained for about 15 min. This will be the picture in a normovolaemic patient.

c. CVP rise by more than 5 cmH$_2$O and is sustained for a longer period indicates probable fluid overload.

CVP is the pressure within the right atrium and great veins of the thorax, usually measured with the patient lying flat. The 'zero' point is the mid-axillary line. CVP is expressed as units of pressure (cmH$_2$O when measuring with a water manometer, mmHg if using an electronic transducer) above this line. By convention, it is measured at end of

27

expiration. The tip of the central venous catheter should ideally lie about 1 cm above the junction of the superior vena cava and right atrium, to reduce the risk of arrhythmias and cardiac tamponade, should erosion occur. The sites that can be used include the internal and external jugular veins in the neck, subclavian vein, femoral vein and veins in the anterior cubital fossa. Arterial puncture, air embolism, pneumothorax and sepsis are some of the major complications of central venous cannulation.

3. *At 1800 h you are called to the Urology ward to assess a postoperative patient who has pulled out his urinary catheter and venous cannula. When you reach the ward, he is demanding to go home and has accused the nurse of stealing his money. He asks you to call the Police. His notes reveal that he had undergone a trans-urethral resection of the prostate (TURP) under spinal anaesthesia that afternoon and the resection took 90 min. He was admitted 3 days earlier as he had gone into acute urinary retention and could not cope alone at home since his wife died 3 months ago.*

Why is he suddenly confused?

The possible causes include hypoxia, hypercapnia, hypotension, hypovolaemia, pain and drugs (especially those that depress the central nervous system and those with central anticholinergic effects caused by lipid soluble drugs like atropine and cyclizine). Metabolic disturbances like hypoglycaemia, hypo- and hypernatraemia, acidosis and withdrawal of alcohol and benzodiazepines should also be considered. Confusion presenting after any procedure that involves irrigating body cavities with a glycine solution (e.g. TURP, trans-urethral resection of bladder tumour (TURBT), or trans-anal resections) may be a result of 'TUR syndrome' (see below).

What is your plan of action?

Your ability to handle volatile situations is put to the test here! Invariably the nursing staff will be at their wits end and might pressurise you to prescribe a sedative. Initiate practical measures to calm and orientate the patient.

Presence of a relative or friend of the patient will be very helpful. Find a well-lit room/place for the patient. In extreme cases you may need to restrain the patient physically with the help of others.

As the cause of the confusion can have so many possibilities, you would like to do a battery of investigations and observations. But practically this can be very challenging. If the confusion is due to hypoxia and/or hypotension, sedation with a major tranquilliser might aggravate the problem. Even administering oxygen by mask will be difficult. In most places, obtaining liaison psychiatric help at this time of the day is a problem.

27

Are any investigations justified or is there any more history that might help?

Try to get a clear picture about the preoperative mental status and social situation of the patient. Look for clues as to alcohol and other drug abuse like recent bereavement and failure to cope at home.

Investigations of importance include:

FBC: to look for anaemia, sepsis.

U&E: detect hypo-osmolality, widened osmolar gap, hyponatraemia, and other electrolyte abnormalities.

ECG: evidence of ischaemia, infarction, electrolyte abnormalities.

ABG: to rule out hypoxia, hypercarbia and acidosis and in fluid overload may show hypoxia with respiratory alkalosis.

Osmolality is an expression of the concentration of osmotically active particles in solution. Osmolality of plasma is maintained between 280–305 mOsm/kg. Most contribution to plasma osmolality arises from sodium and its anions, glucose and urea. Osmolar gap is the difference between calculated and measured plasma osmolality. Normally under 10 mOsm/kg, it is increased by high levels of osmotically active substances, e.g. alcohols, glycine, mannitol.

$$\text{Calculated serum osmolality (mOsm/kg)} = [\text{glucose}] + [\text{urea}] + (2 \times [\text{Na}^+])$$
$$\text{(all in mmol/l)}$$

Here the history does give clues towards alcohol abuse. More importantly, the chances of TUR syndrome are also high. TURP done under spinal with a resection time of 90 min raises the possibility.

Hb	8.9 g/dl
WBC	5.6×10^9/l
Platelets	200×10^9/l
plasma sodium	120 mmol/l
plasma potassium	3.2 mmol/l
plasma urea	5.7 mmol/l
plasma creatinine	100 µmol/l
serum osmolality	265 mOsm/kg
osmolar gap	25 mOsm/kg
Arterial blood gases (ABGs), on air:	
pH	7.48
pCO_2	3.0 kPa
P_aO_2	9.5 kPa
plasma bicarbonate	21.5 mmol/l
base excess	−3.0 mmol/l
S_aO_2	95.5%
ECG	no change since preoperative ECG no evidence of myocardial ischaemia

27

TUR syndrome is caused by absorption of irrigating fluid through open prostatic vessels, usually hypotonic glycine 1.5%. Glycine is used in such procedures as it does not conduct electricity allowing diathermy to tissues. Symptoms are caused by intravascular volume overload, dilutional hyponatraemia and intracellular oedema. Glycine and its metabolites (e.g. ammonia) also have systemic effects. Features include bradycardia, hypotension, angina, dyspnoea, confusion, convulsions and coma. Glycine is also an inhibitory neurotransmitter so confusion or coma may not simply be due to electrolyte imbalance. Severity depends on the volume of fluid absorbed. The amount of fluid absorbed will depend on the pressure of infusion (during the procedure the maximum height of the reservoir bag should be 60 cm above the patient), venous pressure (avoid hypovolaemia and hypotension), duration of resection (limit resection time to <60 min) and the tonicity of irrigating fluid. Use of regional anaesthesia will help respiratory and mental status monitoring and early detection. CVP measurement is helpful in susceptible patients. Intra-operative monitoring of tracer substances like 10% ethanol added to irrigating fluid and measured in breath or blood has been described. Management is that of hyponatraemia, convulsions and raised ICP. Diuretics, hypertonic saline and vasopressors may be required, but such interventions require specialist help and monitoring.

4. *You are the junior doctor on the evening shift covering the surgical wards. A nurse has requested you to review a 50-year-old patient in the postoperative ward with a systolic BP of 90 mmHg. This gentleman had a sigmoid colectomy for diverticular disease 24 h ago. He is a type II diabetic on an insulin sliding scale. His pain is well controlled with an epidural, but he feels rather sick.*

Why do you think he feels so sick?

Important factors causing nausea in this postoperative patient include relative hypotension, hypoglycaemia, pain, GI surgery, ileus, gastric distension and drugs (e.g. opioids).

This patient's last blood sugar was 5.2 mmol/l, measured half an hour ago. He has good pain relief with an epidural infusion. His nasogastric tube is draining freely and has had no systemic opioid for pain relief. His peripheries are warm and well perfused.

Why do you think his BP is so low?

Most common cause of hypotension in the postoperative period includes absolute hypovolaemia and relative hypovolaemia due to epidural block, rewarming, sepsis and anaphylaxis. Other causes especially in the first 24–48 h following surgery are arrhythmias, myocardial ischaemia or infarction, heart failure and pulmonary embolism.

If hypoglycaemia was the cause, airway, breathing and level of consciousness might be affected. Administer oxygen and whilst

27

repeating a finger prick blood glucose quickly assess these, using the AVPU scale for level of consciousness:

A = alert

V = responds to voice

P = responds to pain

U = unresponsive

If the hypoglycaemia was not profound and the patient was alert and able to eat, they could be given a milky drink and a biscuit. Diabetic patients treated with insulin are often very adept at recognising 'hypos', but the normal symptoms and signs can be masked by opioids. So soon after bowel surgery this patient would require 50 ml 50% dextrose IV.

You take blood and send it to the laboratory:

Hb	11.5 g/dl
Hct	0.32
WBC	7.5×10^9/l
Platelets	124×10^9/l
plasma sodium	140 mmol/l
plasma potassium	4.5 mmol/l
plasma urea	7.5 mmol/l
plasma creatinine	113 μmol/l
plasma glucose	5.0 mmol/l
ECG	Sinus tachycardia

It can be very difficult to tell why patients with epidural infusions *in situ* are hypotensive. Local anaesthetic in the epidural infusion blocks not only motor neurons and neurons in the pain pathways, but also sympathetic fibres responsible for maintaining vasomotor tone. Thus epidurals cause vasodilatation and relative hypotension. However, after an operation this is likely to co-exist with dehydration. These investigations and findings reveal the most probable cause of hypotension in this patient is the vasodilatation and relative hypovolaemia due to the epidural block. The clue is that the patient's peripheries are warm and well perfused.

Most hospitals now have an acute pain team to consult regarding the management of these issues during 'office hours'. It is always wise to seek the opinion of the on call anaesthetist out of hours. Monitoring the level of central neuraxial block achieved by the epidural is the key to successful epidural pain management. It is often most appropriate to nurse these patients in a high dependency area with a higher nurse to patient ratio. The nursing staff should regularly check the level of the epidural block with an ice cube and record it. You should remember that usually the level of sympathetic block will be two segments above this and cardiac sympathetic fibres will be affected with blocks above T4.

27

What are you going to do about the hypotension?

Administer high concentration oxygen by mask. Here the concern is of relative intravascular hypovolaemia due to sympathetic block induced vasodilatation. Assess fluid balance over the past 24 h with particular reference to urine output. His kidneys will have developed some amount of diabetic microangiopathy and will require higher mean arterial pressure to maintain adequate glomerular filtration. Consult an anaesthetist or the acute pain team for advice. He probably needs intravenous infusion of fluids.

What is he at risk of?

The end organs affected by diabetic microangiopathy are the brain, heart, kidneys and the gut. The perfusion to these organs becomes dependent on a high mean arterial pressure. Persistent hypoperfusion can precipitate ischaemia and infarction in these vital organs, manifesting as confusion, angina, MI, acute tubular necrosis and ischaemia of the bowel wall, which can contribute to bacterial translocation and sepsis.

5. *You are the Senior House Officer covering orthopaedics tonight. A 97-year-old lady from a nursing home is suddenly very wheezy after an Austin Moore hemiarthroplasty under spinal anaesthesia that afternoon. She is demented, nobody has made the effort to take a proper history or contact the GP since she fractured her hip. She is fighting for breath and rather agitated, asking for help.*

Differential diagnosis of postoperative breathlessness and wheezing includes pulmonary oedema, acute exacerbation of chronic obstructive pulmonary disease, pneumonia and pulmonary embolus. This highlights the importance of obtaining a proper history. In a patient with preexisting wheeze, pneumothorax should also be considered.

What do you do straight away?

Always remember the A, B, and C of resuscitation. Here we can assume that the airway is patent as she is speaking. First sit her up and give oxygen by mask. Ask the nurse if she could kindly obtain as much past medical history as possible from the GP or nursing home. Review her observations chart since admission and return from theatre and look for any clues. Conduct a thorough general and systemic examination.

Administering high concentration oxygen to patients with chronic obstructive pulmonary disease (COPD) always causes great anxiety amongst medical, nursing and paramedical staff. Only a minority of patients with chronic obstructive pulmonary disease who retain CO_2 rely on hypoxaemia for respiratory drive and can be rendered apnoeic by high oxygen concentrations. The majority of patients with chronic lung disease are under treated with oxygen for this reason. Carefully monitoring respiratory rate and regular ABGs will detect the onset of hypercapnoea under these circumstances.

27

The nurse comes back and tells you that this patient had a heart attack 10 years ago, takes aspirin and ramipril and is not thought to have a history of lung disease. At the Home she was mobile with a frame but very frail. The Nursing Home staff cannot remember her complaining of chest pain.

Preoperative observations:

Heart rate	88/min
Blood pressure	170/90 mmHg
Respiratory rate	17/min
Core temperature	35.8°C

Immediate postoperative observations:

Heart rate	86/min
Blood pressure	120/75 mmHg
Respiratory rate	24/min
Core temperature	36.4°C

Postoperative observations after 8 h:

Heart rate	111/min
Blood pressure	110/70 mmHg
Respiratory rate	34/min
Core temperature	35.5°C

27

What are the salient points in the examination and how can they help you to make a diagnosis?

During examination look for clues to diagnosis: cold extremities, cyanosis, raised JVP, rapid thready pulse, noisy breathing, dull percussion note at bases, absence of air entry, type of breath sounds, basal air entry, presence of crepitations and rhonchi, etc. Presence or absence of any of these findings will help to make a diagnosis of acute left ventricular failure (LVF), pneumonia, acute exacerbation of asthma or COPD. Remember that wheeze is caused by narrow airways. Do not automatically assume that a patient with a wheezy chest has asthma or COPD, airways are narrowed by bronchospasm but also when they fill with fluid so LVF should always be a differential diagnosis. Even if there is a loud wheeze in the chest, consider how unusual it would be for a 97-year-old lady to have an asthma attack out of the blue! If you cannot distinguish between early pulmonary oedema, asthma or pneumonia, treat for all three. If there are no signs of LVF or asthma, consider PE.

On examination:

Heart rate	118/min
Blood pressure	110/60 mmHg
Respiratory rate	36/min
Oral temperature	36.3°C

The peripheries are cold and clammy; JVP is visible 6 cm above the clavicle, air entry is reduced at both lung bases, widespread fine crepitations and rhonchi are heard.

Is there any other information at the bedside that can help you?

Here you are looking for evidence of fluid overload leading to acute LVF. Any information regarding fluid input and output during the last 24–48 h will be valuable. Look into the fluid balance chart, fluid prescription chart, anaesthetic chart and drugs brought in from the nursing home.

Fluid balance chart:

Fluid input	'Oral intake' written on chart but quantity not documented
Urine output	Has been wetting the bed and is not yet catheterised

Fluid prescription chart:

- 5% dextrose 1,000 ml over 10 h × 2 given preoperatively
- 0.9% saline 1,000 ml over 10 h × 2 prescribed postoperatively, of which about 800 ml has been given

Anaesthetic chart:

- Intra-operative fluids given were Hartmann's 1,000 ml, Gelofusine 1,000 ml
- Ephedrine 3 mg × 3 doses

What investigations would help?

FBC: may reveal haemodilution, sepsis.

U&E: non-specific, but may reveal underlying compromised renal function.

27

ABGs: hypoxia, hypocarbia, acidosis. $P_a\text{co}_2$ is usually at low end of normal, but this might be lower if PE is suspected.

CXR: might be helpful, but differentiating pulmonary oedema from early pneumonia is difficult. A baseline for comparison will be helpful.

ECG: this should be compared with the preoperative baseline ECG to assess whether there is a new arrhythmia, worsening myocardial ischaemia or myocardial infarction.

What is going on here?

This lady has acute left ventricular failure, brought on by fluid overload, myocardial ischaemia or both. The spinal block she received in theatre blocks sympathetic nerve fibres just like an epidural, causing vasodilatation and relative hypovolaemia. The block is more intense with a spinal and wears off after approximately 1.5–2 h. When vasomotor tone is restored, fluid overload can occur and patients with little or no cardiac reserve can develop LVF.

What should be done next?

Sit this lady up, continue oxygen and make an emergency referral to the on call medical team. They are likely to move her to a Coronary Care or High Dependency Unit and administer opioids, vasodilators and diuretics.

6. *You are the Senior House Officer in the Accident and Emergency Department. A motorcyclist sustained an open fracture of the left tibia and fibula and open book pelvic fracture 2 h ago and is waiting to go to theatre. He is receiving his fourth unit of blood which restored his blood pressure initially, but suddenly it is unrecordable. You are alone with him, as the trauma team have been called to another emergency.*

What is your immediate action?

Always remember A, B and C. Assessment of airway, breathing and circulation is done whilst calling for help. Maintain the airway and give 100% oxygen. If he is not breathing you can use a bag-valve-mask unit to ventilate him. In the absence of a pulse, chest compressions should be commenced. Ask the nurse to connect the ECG leads of the defibrillator machine and examine the ECG rhythm strip.

No breathing movements noted and you could not feel a carotid pulse!

ECG   sinus rhythm

This is a picture of EMD arrest.

You notice that the patient has large red blotches all over his body and a swollen face. What is going on?

Transfusion reaction. This is a very difficult but vital diagnosis to make. Skin changes are not that common during a transfusion reaction. In this case it could be easy to imagine that there is suddenly catastrophic internal haemorrhage and you would treat this by speeding up the blood transfusion.

27

251

What is the management of this medical emergency?

STOP THE TRANSFUSION IMMEDIATELY. Ensure that help is on its way. Remove the bag and giving set and send it to the lab later. Commence cardiopulmonary resuscitation. This patient is already likely to have wide bore IV access. Give 1 mg (10 ml of 1:10,000) adrenaline (epinephrine) as per the Resuscitation Council protocol. Also start fluid replacement (probably colloids). At an appropriate time, intubation is necessary followed by ventilation with 100% oxygen. Once pulse pressure returns the circulation is likely to need support with further adrenaline (epinephrine) in 50 mcg IV increments (0.5 ml of 1:10,000 solution) at a rate of 100 mcg/min. The anaesthetist/intensive care physician is likely to start an adrenaline (epinephrine) infusion before transfer to the intensive care unit. Subsequent management involves antihistamines, corticosteroids and inotrope infusions for cardiovascular stability. Check ABGs for metabolic acidosis, which may require bicarbonate for correction. Consider bronchodilators if there is persistent bronchospasm. Investigations can wait until the patient has been stabilised. Take a 10 ml clotted blood sample 1 h after the episode to perform a tryptase assay.

Arterial blood gases (ABGs), on 100% O_2:

pH	7.15
P_aCO_2	5.6 kPa
P_aO_2	18.4 kPa
plasma bicarbonate	15.7 mmol/l
base excess	−8.9 mmol/l
S_aO_2	99.5%

27

Although the P_aO_2 seems to be well above the normal range, it is far from satisfactory as the patient is ventilated with 100% oxygen. There is a simple equation that allows you to quantify how appropriate a patient's P_aO_2 is, whilst taking into account the concentration of inspired oxygen. It is the P_aO_2/F_iO_2 ratio (where P_aO_2 is the partial pressure of oxygen in arterial blood and F_iO_2 is the fraction of inspired oxygen expressed as a fraction of 1):

A normal person breathing air:

$$\frac{P_aO_2}{F_iO_2} = \frac{12}{0.21} = \text{approximately } 60$$

Air is 21% oxygen so the F_iO_2 is 0.21. So you can see that when gas exchange is normal, P_aO_2 increases with F_iO_2, and the ratio will stay the same.

This patient is on 100% oxygen:

$$\frac{P_aO_2}{F_IO_2} = \frac{18.4}{1.0} = 18.4$$

As gas exchange deteriorates, the $P_aO_2{:}F_IO_2$ ratio falls. The ratio is a useful way of monitoring the efficacy of treatment for acute respiratory emergencies. For example, imagine that a young man with acute severe asthma presents to Accident and Emergency:

Initial blood gases, F_IO_2 0.50:

pH	7.20	(NR: 7.35–7.45)
P_aCO_2	3.6 kPa	(NR: 4.5–6.0)
P_aO_2	9.5 kPa	(NR: ≥11.0)
plasma bicarbonate	16.5 mmol/l	(NR: 21–28)
base excess	−7.1 mmol/l	(NR: −2–+2)
S_aO_2	96.5%	

He has a metabolic acidosis with respiratory compensation. You calculate the $P_aO_2{:}F_IO_2$ ratio to be 19. You start treatment but are distracted by another emergency. Fifteen minutes later you are shown a new set of blood gases. Now he is breathing 100% oxygen via a face mask: At first glance the ABG results are satisfying, as both P_aO_2 and P_aCO_2 now lie within the normal range. However, the $P_aO_2{:}F_IO_2$ ratio has fallen to 11.5. Gas exchange has actually deteriorated. This is reflected by the worsening acidosis.

pH	7.13	(NR: 7.35–7.45)
P_aCO_2	4.5 kPa	(NR: 4.5–6.0)
P_aO_2	11.5 kPa	(NR: ≥11.0)
plasma bicarbonate	15.1 mmol/l	(NR: 21–28)
base excess	−8.9 mmol/l	(NR: −2–+2)
S_aO_2	97.0%	

27

Interpreting ABG results is no substitute for clinical assessment of a patient, but if you had not calculated the $P_aO_2{:}F_IO_2$ ratio you might have been lulled into thinking that the treatment was working. Examining this patient now you would find that he is in extremis, on the verge of respiratory arrest with falling respiratory rate and tidal volume, accounting for the increased P_aco_2.

This additional scenario highlights four important points:

1. Always treat the patient, not the results.

2. Results that lie within the normal range do not necessarily represent normality and should be seen as part of a trend.

3. ABG results are worthless unless accompanied by a record of the F_io_2 at the time the sample was taken.

4. As the F_io_2 delivered by variable performance oxygen masks is difficult to quantify, oxygen should be delivered via a fixed performance mask with a Venturi valve to patients with acute respiratory emergencies.

(See also the Chapter 16: Arterial blood gases)

7. *You are asked to go and sort out the pain of a 9-year-old boy in Accident and Emergency. He has been complaining of right iliac fossa pain and the surgeons believe it is an inflamed appendix. He is due for theatre when one is available. He has a history of mild asthma.*

What are your thoughts on the way down to casualty?

Revise the chapter on perioperative pain management! Think of the options you have and indications and contra-indications for each of those choices. Think of a method to assess the severity of his pain. Remember the principle of multimodal approach.

Assuming he has an appendicectomy, what pain relief will you prescribe pre- and postoperatively?

Paracetamol and NSAIDs are widely prescribed for this type of pain. They have an opioid sparing effect as well. History of mild asthma alone does not necessarily contra-indicate the use of NSAIDs. Many children have a wheezy episode at some stage and may be prescribed an inhaler. This does not necessary mean they have asthma! To deny all children who have an inhaler in the home NSAIDs would be to deny a large group a reliable and useful analgesic. Ask a parent if the child has ever taken ibuprofen elixir (many trade names, e.g. Nurofen for children®) without complication. Some patients or parents may report that they have been told never to take NSAIDs due to their asthma. If this is the case, ask who told them this. It may have been a pharmacist selling an over-the-counter NSAID preparation who might have an over cautious attitude and does not have the time to take a full history.

There are asthmatics in whom severe bronchospasm can be precipitated by NSAIDs. They tend to be young, brittle asthmatics with nasal polyposis, and will often give you a history. If in doubt prescribing NSAIDs to asthmatics, ask a colleague.

This child does not give any history suggestive of nasal polyps, has had only mild asthmatic attacks and was never hospitalised during any of these attacks.

What are the doses of important analgesics, and what is your preferred route of administration?

The preferred routes of administration in children are oral and rectal. You will be unpopular with children, parents and nurses alike if you prescribed intramuscular analgesics without a VERY good reason!

Suggested doses of analgesics for perioperative pain in children. In children less than 1 year old, ask an anaesthesist or paediatrician for advice.

Drug	By age	By weight
Paracetamol	Oral: 1–5 yrs: 120–250 mg up to 4 times a day 6–12 yrs: 250–500 mg up to 4 times a day 12 yrs +: 500–1000 mg up to 4 times a day Same doses rectally	Loading dose: 30 mg/kg once rectally then: 10–15 mg/kg up to 4 times a day, rectally or orally
Ibuprofen	1–2 yrs: 50 mg 3–4 times a day orally 3–7 yrs : 100 mg 3–4 times a day orally 8–12 yrs : 200 mg 3–4 times a day orally 12 yrs +: 200–400 mg 3–4 times a day orally	20–30 mg/kg in divided doses orally
Diclofenac sodium		1–16 yrs: 1–3 mg/kg in 2 or 3 divided doses orally or rectally, not intramuscularly
Codeine phosphate		1–16 yrs: 1 mg/kg in divided doses, orally, rectally (or intramuscularly)
Morphine sulphate		1–16 yrs: 0.1 mg/kg orally (intramuscularly) Seek help before prescribing intravenously

27

What are the side effects of the drugs you have prescribed?

Paracetamol: usually very well tolerated, as has minimal anti-inflammatory action. Does not cause gastric irritation or alter platelet function. It may cause hepatic necrosis in poisoning. Use is limited to <5 days continuously.

NSAIDs: by their effect on prostaglandin metabolism, they can affect platelet function and cause bleeding, bronchial smooth muscle contraction leading to acute exacerbation of asthma, destruction of gastric mucosal barrier causing gastric bleeding and acute tubular necrosis with renal failure. Never prescribe aspirin to a child under 12 years, as it can precipitate Reye's syndrome (hepatic failure and cerebral oedema). This guideline may soon be altered to include all children under 16.

Opioid: nausea, vomiting, itching, respiratory depression, bradycardia, hypotension, urinary retention, euphoria and dysphoria, dry mouth, blurred vision.

27

28

Multiple choice questions

Quentin Milner

Each question has four stems. Answer true or false for each statement. A correct answer scores $+1$, an incorrect answer scores -1 and no answer scores 0.

There are three different exams.

Exams 1 and 2 consist of 30 questions and should take 30 min to complete.

Exam 3 has only 10 questions for a quick fire test.

Exam 1

1. Pulse oximetry
a. pulse oximeters measure the amount of oxygen dissolved in blood.
b. readings over 75% are normal.
c. patients with S_pO_2 >90% should not receive supplemental oxygen as this may depress respiratory drive.
d. is not affected by skin pigmentation.

2. The following occur commonly in the early postoperative period
a. shivering.
b. hypertension.
c. unilateral weakness.
d. hyperthermia.

3. In the event of intubation of the right main bronchus, the following would occur within the next 10 min
a. increased requirement for volatile anaesthetic agent.
b. hypoxaemia.
c. decreased ventilatory pressures.
d. a rise in arterial CO_2 tension.

4. When prescribing postoperative fluids you should
a. disregard patient's temperature.
b. prescribe 1 litre of normal saline each day.
c. only prescribe potassium supplements for patients in renal failure.
d. repeat what was prescribed in theatre.

5. As a surgical houseman you are called to see an elderly patient who is confused postoperatively. Which of the following statements are true?
a. confusion in the elderly is common and can be accepted for up to 4 h postoperatively whilst anaesthetic drugs are being metabolised.
b. hypotension is a common cause of confusion.
c. hypoxia is unlikely to be the cause.
d. you should immediately do an arterial blood gas sample.

28

6. Patient controlled analgesia devices
a. are suitable for any type of analgesic.
b. are safer than continuous infusion of opioids.
c. can be reprogrammed by patients themselves if they are not providing adequate analgesia.
d. can prevent the patient from suffering nausea and vomiting post operatively.

7. The minimum alveolar concentration (MAC) of a volatile anaesthetic agent
a. is the minimum vaporiser concentration setting required to know that a patient is asleep.
b. is the same for everybody, regardless of age.
c. depends on sex.
d. depends on age.

8. Nitrous oxide (N_2O)
a. allows less oxygen to be administered to the patient.
b. cannot be used with intravenous anaesthetic agents.
c. is an anaesthetic agent.
d. can only be delivered by a doctor.

9. A sensible postoperative dose of morphine for a 70 kg adult after intermediate surgery would be
a. 0.1 mg IM every 4 h.
b. 1.0 mg IM every 4 h.
c. 10 mg IM every 4 h.
d. 100 mg IM every 4 h.

10. Recognised side effects of morphine are
a. nausea and vomiting.
b. hallucinations.
c. itching.
d. respiratory depression.

11. Management of a patient who has received an overdose of morphine from a patient controlled analgesia (PCA) machine includes
a. immediate supplemental oxygen.
b. immediate intubation and ventilation.
c. intravenous naloxone.
d. reduction of the PCA machine to continuous infusion mode.

28

12. Patient controlled analgesia (PCA) devices
a. can be used by all patients once they have been shown how to use them.
b. are safe for nurses to prescribe.
c. can only be used in high dependency units.
d. must always have lockout periods in them.

13. Patient controlled analgesia devices
a. record the amount of analgesic agent given to the patient.
b. remove the need to provide other types of analgesia postoperatively.
c. require a functioning intravenous cannula and one way valve.
d. are suitable for all types of operation.

14. Patients suspected of having a serious anaphylactic reaction to a drug
a. should be given high flow oxygen by facemask.
b. should not receive adrenaline (epinephrine) as this may cause arrhythmias.
c. should have an intravenous drip inserted and be given IV fluids.
d. may also have reactions to other totally different drugs.

15. Concerning anaphylaxis
a. patients will always have bronchospasm and wheeze.
b. adrenaline (epinephrine) is the drug of choice if hypotension is present.
c. oxygen should only be given if hypoxia has been demonstrated on a blood gas.
d. anaphylaxis cannot occur without a rash appearing.

16. The differential diagnosis of a patient with hypotension following induction of anaesthesia includes
a. hypovolaemia.
b. dehydration.
c. overdose of an anaesthetic agent.
d. malignant hyperpyrexia.

17. An obese patient is more likely to be
a. difficult to intubate.
b. hypoxaemic.
c. hypercarbic postoperatively.
d. hypertensive.

18. The following statements about postoperative fluid balance are correct
a. patients given large amounts of fluid in theatre will need less fluid in the postoperative phase.
b. adequate urine output is above 0.5 ml/kg/h.
c. an average sized patient needs 3 litres of water per day.
d. dextrose carries enough calories to meet daily energy requirements.

19. Normal daily requirements of electrolytes are
a. sodium 1–2 mmol/kg.
b. potassium 1–2 mmol/kg.
c. zinc 1–2 mmol/kg.
d. calcium 1–2 mmol/kg.

28

20. Regarding intravenous fluids
a. postoperative fluid prescriptions should be made in theatre for the succeeding 3 days.
b. inadvertent intravenous injection of air will only be life threatening in the presence of a ventricular septal defect.
c. inadvertent intravenous injection of air will only be life threatening in the presence of atrial septal defect.
d. will usually not cause problems unless more than 50 ml is injected.

21. Fluid losses during surgery can be caused by
a. blood loss.
b. hypothermia.
c. evaporation.
d. radiation.

22. Blood transfusion should be considered for a patient when
a. the patient's Hb is less than 12 g/dl.
b. when more than 5% of the blood volume has been lost.
c. when more than 10% of the blood volume has been lost.
d. when more than 400 ml of blood has been lost.

23. The following statements about suxamethonium are correct
a. suxamethonium is metabolised in the liver.
b. suxamethonium can cause muscular pains following injection.
c. suxamethonium causes the release of intracellular potassium.
d. caution should be exercised when giving suxamethonium to pregnant women.

24. Indications for endotracheal intubation during anaesthesia include
a. alcohol intoxication.
b. HIV infection.
c. active TB.
d. small bowel obstruction.

25. The following statements concerning fluids and electrolytes are correct
a. 70% of the body mass is water in an adult male.
b. 80% of the body mass of a neonate is water.
c. potassium is largely an extracellular electrolyte.
d. calcium is largely an intracellular electrolyte.

28

26. Heat loss during anaesthesia is caused by
a. conduction.
b. convection.
c. evaporation.
d. decreased metabolic activity.

27. Signs of fluid overload in a patient include
a. palmar erythema.
b. gallop rhythm.
c. tachypnoea.
d. decreased central venous pressure.

28. The following devices protect the airway from soiling in an anaesthetised patient:
a. laryngeal mask airway.
b. cuffed endotracheal tube.
c. guedel airway.
d. nasogastric tube.

29. Endobronchial intubation is
a. more common in adults than children.
b. more common in men than women.
c. more common in the right main bronchus than left main bronchus.
d. more common in patients breathing spontaneously.

30. In a normal subject cardiac output is increased by
a. pyrexia.
b. increased CVP.
c. increase in heart rate.
d. increase in metabolic rate.

Answers Exam 1

1. a. F
    b. F
    c. F
    d. T

2. a. T
    b. F
    c. F
    d. F

3. a. T
    b. T
    c. F
    d. T

4. a. F
    b. F
    c. F
    d. F

5. a. F
    b. T
    c. F
    d. F

6. a. F
    b. T
    c. F
    d. F

7. a. F
    b. F
    c. F
    d. T

8. a. F
    b. F
    c. T
    d. F

9. a. F
    b. F
    c. T
    d. F

10. a. T
    b. T
    c. T
    d. T

11. a. T
    b. F
    c. T
    d. F

12. a. T
    b. F
    c. F
    d. T

13. a. T
    b. F
    c. T
    d. F

14. a. T
    b. F
    c. T
    d. T

28

15. a. F
    b. T
    c. F
    d. F

16. a. T
    b. T
    c. T
    d. F

17. a. T
    b. T
    c. T
    d. T

18. a. F
    b. T
    c. T
    d. F

19. a. T
    b. T
    c. F
    d. F

20. a. F
    b. F
    c. F
    d. F

21. a. T
    b. F
    c. T
    d. F

22. a. F
    b. F
    c. T
    d. F

23. a. F
    b. T
    c. T
    d. F

24. a. T
    b. F
    c. F
    d. T

28

25. a. T
    b. T
    c. F
    d. F

26. a. T
    b. T
    c. T
    d. F

27. a. F
    b. T
    c. T
    d. F

28. a. F
    b. T
    c. F
    d. F

29. a. T
    b. F
    c. T
    d. F

30. a. T
    b. T
    c. T
    d. T

Exam 2

1. Appropriate drugs to use for a rapid sequence induction include
a. Propofol.
b. Thiopentone.
c. Atracurium.
d. Suxamethonium.

2. Myocardial contractility is influenced by
a. Plasma potassium concentration.
b. Heart rate.
c. Circulating volume.
d. Parasympathetic nervous system activity.

28

3. After the inhalation of gastric contents the following may occur
a. Hypoxia.
b. Hypovolaemia.
c. Hypercarbia.
d. Hypotension.

4. In an elective patient which of the following require investigation before anaesthesia?
a. Diastolic blood pressure of 115 mmHg.
b. Systolic blood pressure of 160 mmHg.
c. Mean arterial blood pressure (MAP) of 50 mmHg.
d. Central venous pressure of 6 mmHg.

5. Prolonged vomiting can cause
a. Haematemesis.
b. Hyperchloraemia.
c. Metabolic alkalosis.
d. Hypokalaemia.

6. Complications of massive blood transfusion include
a. Hypothermia.
b. Hyperkalaemia.
c. Hyponatraemia.
d. Hyperalbuminaemia.

7. P waves are absent from the ECG in the following conditions
a. Thyrotoxicosis.
b. Atrial fibrillation.
c. Supraventricular tachycardia.
d. Complete heart block.

8. With regard to ABO blood groups
a. Group O is found in 60% of the population.
b. Group AB patients have antibodies to both A and B groups.
c. A full cross match achieves compatibility in 99.95% of cases.
d. Giving unmatched blood will achieve compatibility in 60% of cases.

9. When assessing a patient with asthma preoperatively
a. Pulmonary function may vary during the day.
b. An elevated PCO_2 is a common finding.
c. The chest X-ray is an essential investigation.
d. The ECG will be normal in all but those with severe disease.

10. Which of the following statements about intravenous fluids are correct
a. When replacing blood with crystalloids three times the volume of blood lost should be given.

b. A litre of normal saline will be distributed equally throughout the intracellular and extracellular volumes.

c. A litre of 5% dextrose will be distributed equally throughout the intracellular and extracellular volumes.

d. Some types of colloid solutions are made from purified beef extracts.

11. Signs of ischaemic heart disease include
a. Gallop rhythm.
b. Raised JVP.
c. Pulsus alternans.
d. Decreased cardiothoracic ratio.

12. The following may be present in chronic obstructive pulmonary disease (COPD)
a. Palpable liver edge.
b. Clubbing.
c. Cyanosis.
d. Decreased area of cardiac dullness on percussion.

13. Immediately following sudden massive haemorrhage there will be
a. A fall in CVP.
b. Wide spread vasoconstriction.
c. A shift in the oxyhaemoglobin curve to the right.
d. A fall in urine output.

14. In an elective patient, which of the following should be corrected prior to anaesthesia?
a. First degree heart block.
b. Plasma glucose of 6.5 mmol/l.
c. Haemoglobin concentration of 11 g/dl.
d. Plasma potassium concentration of 2.5 mmol/l.

15. Nitrous oxide (N_2O)
a. Is an analgesic agent as well as an anaesthetic agent.
b. Should never be given to pregnant women in the first stage of labour.
c. Can be given to women in labour with 50% air.
d. Can only be used in patients connected to a ventilator.

16. Volatile anaesthetic agents are
a. Better than intravenous anaesthetic agents at ensuring a patient is asleep.
b. Always used in an anaesthetic.
c. Never used for people with ischaemic heart disease.
d. Inflammable.

28

17. Intravenous anaesthetic agents
a. Induce anaesthesia faster than inhalational anaesthetics.
b. Can be painful on injection.
c. Provide all the analgesia required in an operation.
d. Are all water soluble.

18. Most life threatening complications of anaesthesia tend to occur
a. During the induction of anaesthesia.
b. During maintenance of anaesthesia.
c. During emergence from anaesthesia.
d. In the recovery area.

19. Concerning morphine prescribed for postoperative pain relief
a. Any patient who is sleepy but still in pain should not have more morphine for fear of overdose.
b. Morphine should only be used for postoperative pain if it has not been used intra-operatively.
c. Naloxone is the antagonist to morphine overdose.
d. Morphine has less analgesic properties than midazolam.

20. Clinical signs of a tension pneumothorax under anaesthesia are
a. Hypotension.
b. Tracheal shift to the side of the pneumothorax.
c. Decreased breath sounds on the side of the pneumothorax.
d. Increased JVP.

21. Concerning postoperative nausea and vomiting, which of the following statements are true?
a. Women are affected more than men.
b. Middle ear surgery is commonly associated with nausea and vomiting.
c. If one anti-emetic has been unsuccessful, a different class of anti-emetic should be prescribed.
d. Children are very rarely sick after anaesthesia.

22. When a patient with asthma is scheduled for theatre
a. He should be started on oral steroids one week prior to the date of operation.
b. He should always have a preoperative chest X-ray.
c. He should have his peak flow checked on admission to the ward.
d. He should continue his normal medications on the day of surgery.

23. Common clinical findings in ischaemic heart disease are
a. Increased cardiothoracic ratio.
b. A history of intermittent claudication.
c. A mid-diastolic murmur.
d. Deviation of the ECG axis to the left.

24. Preoperative investigations of a patient with severe COAD include
a. ECG.
b. Arterial blood gases.
c. Plasma bicarbonate.
d. FEV_1/FVC ratio.

28

25. Concerning the resuscitation of a patient with ventricular fibrillation

a. Cardiac compressions given well can achieve a cardiac output equivalent to normal.
b. Adrenaline (epinephrine) is the first line treatment.
c. Defibrillation should not be delayed whilst the patient is being intubated.
d. The first defibrillation should be at 200 J.

26. In chronic obstructive pulmonary disease a 'pink puffer' is characterised by

a. A high FEV_1.
b. Central cyanosis.
c. An increased functional residual volume.
d. A flatter oxyhaemoglobin dissociation curve.

27. The following physiological statements are correct

a. The normal adult female Hb concentration is 12–14 g/dl.
b. The normal adult cardiac output is about 5 l/min.
c. The normal adult cardiac stroke volume is about 80 ml.
d. Starling's law does not apply to the heart of an anaesthetised patient.

28. Contra-indications to NSAIDs include

a. Patients receiving haemodialysis.
b. Platelet count less than 200.
c. Patients receiving IV morphine.
d. Patients receiving paracetamol.

29. Signs of hypovolaemia in a patient include

a. Shivering.
b. Confusion.
c. Tachypnoea.
d. Bradycardia.

30. Hypertension in the early postoperative period may be caused by

a. Hypocapnia.
b. Surgical pain.
c. Volatile anaesthetic agents.
d. Full bladder.

28

Answers Exam 2

1. a. T
   b. T
   c. F
   d. T

2. a. F
   b. F
   c. T
   d. T

3. a. T
   b. F
   c. T
   d. T

4. a. T
   b. F
   c. T
   d. F

5. a. T
   b. F
   c. T
   d. T

6. a. T
   b. T
   c. F
   d. F

7. a. F
   b. T
   c. F
   d. F

8. a. F
   b. F
   c. T
   d. T

9. a. T
   b. F
   c. F
   d. T

10. a. T
    b. F
    c. T
    d. T

11. a. F
    b. F
    c. F
    d. F

28

12. a. T
    b. T
    c. T
    d. T

13. a. T
    b. T
    c. F
    d. T

14. a. F
    b. F
    c. F
    d. T

15. a. T
    b. F
    c. F
    d. F

16. a. F
    b. F
    c. F
    d. F

17. a. T
    b. T
    c. F
    d. F

18. a. T
    b. F
    c. T
    d. F

19. a. F
    b. F
    c. T
    d. F

20. a. T
    b. F
    c. T
    d. T

21. a. T
    b. T
    c. T
    d. F

28

22. a. F
    b. F
    c. T
    d. T

23. a. F
    b. F
    c. F
    d. T

24. a. T
    b. T
    c. T
    d. T

25. a. F
    b. F
    c. T
    d. T

26. a. F
    b. F
    c. F
    d. F

27. a. T
    b. T
    c. T
    d. F

28. a. T
    b. F
    c. F
    d. F

29. a. T
    b. T
    c. T
    d. F

30. a. F
    b. T
    c. F
    d. T

Exam 3

1. Naloxone may be used to reverse respiratory depression caused by
a. Pethidine.
b. Codeine.
c. Epidural fentanyl.
d. Thiopentone.

2. Pulmonary oedema may be caused by
a. Tricuspid incompetence.
b. Aortic sclerosis.
c. Myocardial infarction.
d. Mitral incompetence.

3. Defibrillation may be used to treat
a. Asystole.
b. Multifocal ventricular ectopics.
c. Ventricular tachycardia.
d. Pulseless electrical activity (PEA).

4. Patients with sickle cell disease who present for anaesthesia
a. Should receive supplementary oxygen postoperatively.
b. Have a decreased requirement for postoperative analgesia.
c. Have a decreased requirement for perioperative fluids.
d. Should not have a tourniquet applied during surgery.

5. The following drugs may be used to induce anaesthesia
a. Thiopentone.
b. Suxamethonium.
c. Midazolam.
d. Ketamine.

6. Regarding anaemia
a. Anaemia is a common cause of low saturation recorded by a pulse oximeter during anaesthesia.
b. Anaemia is associated with a decreased tissue oxygen delivery when the haematocrit is 0.3.
c. Anaemia is likely to be better tolerated in a patient with chronic renal failure than one with an acute gastro-intestinal haemorrhage.
d. When acute anaemia is corrected by blood transfusion, diuretics should be prescribed with each unit of blood.

7. When resuscitating a patient with burns
a. Analgesic requirements may be high.
b. The patient should be kept cool to dissipate thermal energy.

28

c. Blood transfusion is rarely required for burns below 70% body surface area.

d. Adherence to a protocol for fluid replacement is likely to prevent inadequate fluid administration.

8. The following are recognised risk factors for a perioperative myocardial infarction

a. Presence of a third heart sound.

b. Sinus arrhythmia.

c. Previous CVA.

d. Cardiac ejection fraction of 60%.

9. Which of the following statements are true?

a. Patients graded ASA I have mild systemic diseases which are completely controlled by therapy.

b. Patients graded ASA II have moderate systemic illnesses which are completely controlled by therapy.

c. Patients graded ASA III have severe systemic illnesses which pose a constant threat to life.

d. Patients graded ASA V are moribund and are likely to die with or without surgery.

10. Concerning inotropes

a. Adrenaline (epinephrine) stimulates both alpha and beta receptors.

b. Noradrenaline (norepinephrine) increases the myocardial oxygen demand.

c. Dopexamine stimulates beta-2 receptors.

d. Dobutamine is normally present in the body.

Answers Exam 3

1. a. T
   b. T
   c. T
   d. F

2. a. F
   b. F
   c. T
   d. T

3. a. F
   b. F
   c. T
   d. F

4. a. T
   b. F
   c. F
   d. T

5. a. T
   b. F
   c. T
   d. T

6. a. F
   b. F
   c. T
   d. F

7. a. T
   b. F
   c. F
   d. T

8. a. T
   b. F
   c. T
   d. F

9. a. F
   b. F
   c. F
   d. T

10. a. T
    b. T
    c. T
    d. F

28

Index

Note: 'f' after a page number indicates a reference to a figure, 't' indicates a reference to a table.